Designing Compassion in Hospice Care

Designing Compassion in Hospice Care

The Quiet Room

CHRISTOPHER M. SMITH, RN
Founder and Executive Director,
Freedom Fields Senior Community

OXFORD
UNIVERSITY PRESS

OXFORD
UNIVERSITY PRESS

Oxford University Press is a department of the University of Oxford.
It furthers the University's objective of excellence in research, scholarship,
and education by publishing worldwide. Oxford is a registered trade mark of
Oxford University Press in the UK and in certain other countries.

Published in the United States of America by Oxford University Press
546 Fifth Avenue, New York, NY 10036, United States of America.

Library of Congress Cataloging-in-Publication Data
Names: Smith, Christopher M. (Hospice director) author
Title: Designing compassion in hospice care : the quiet room /
Christopher M. Smith, RN, Clinical Director, Swan Hospice.
Description: New York, NY : Oxford University Press, [2026] | Includes index.
Identifiers: LCCN 2026016599 (print) | LCCN 2026016600 (ebook) |
ISBN 9780197860175 paperback | ISBN 9780197860182 | ISBN 9780197860205 |
ISBN 9780197860199 epub
Subjects: LCSH: Hospice care | Compassion
Classification: LCC R726.8 .S588 2026 (print) | LCC R726.8 (ebook)
LC record available at https://lccn.loc.gov/2026016599
LC ebook record available at https://lccn.loc.gov/2026016600

DOI: 10.1093/med/9780197860175.001.0001

Printed by Marquis Book Printing, Canada

The manufacturer's authorized representative in the EU for product safety is
Oxford University Press España S.A. of El Parque Empresarial San Fernando de Henares,
Avenida de Castilla, 2 – 28830 Madrid (www.oup.es/en or product.safety@oup.com).
OUP España S.A. also acts as importer into Spain of products made by the manufacturer.

FSC
www.fsc.org
MIX
Paper | Supporting
responsible forestry
FSC® C103567

Contents

Preface vii
Acknowledgments ix
Prologue xi

1. The Architecture of Stillness 1
2. The Emotional Architecture of Light 18
3. Objects as Anchors of Presence 34
4. Rituals of Comfort and Continuity 51
5. The Room as Archive 65
6. A Blueprint for the Quiet Room of the Future 79
7. Soundscapes and Acoustic Design 93
8. Olfactory Design in Hospice 108
9. Invisible Tools for Comfort 124
10. Education, Staff Training, and Design Translation 138

Epilogue 153
References 157
Index 161

Preface

This book was born from rooms that rarely announce themselves. They do not call attention through grandeur or spectacle, nor do they demand explanation. They exist at the edges of life's most profound moments, holding space for endings, reckonings, tenderness, and presence. These rooms—often called quiet rooms, comfort rooms, or vigil spaces—are where people arrive when words fail and time feels suspended.

I have stood in these rooms as a caregiver, a witness, and a participant in moments that cannot be hurried or undone. Over time, it became clear that what happens in these spaces is shaped not only by the people within them but also by the architecture itself. Light, sound, texture, and spatial arrangement quietly influence how grief unfolds, how love is expressed, and how dignity is preserved at the end of life.

This book is not a manual in the traditional sense. It does not offer rigid formulas or prescriptive layouts meant to standardize something as intimate as death. Instead, it is an exploration of how space participates in care—how rooms listen, respond, and sometimes even teach. It asks what happens when design is approached not as decoration or efficiency but, rather, as an ethical act.

Hospice work reveals truths that are easy to overlook elsewhere. It strips away pretense and exposes what people need most when everything else falls away: safety, presence, permission, and time. In these moments, the room itself becomes an active companion. It can either support the emotional weight of the moment or quietly undermine it.

Throughout this book, architecture is treated not as background but as a living framework that holds human experience. Chairs become invitations. Light becomes language. Silence becomes a form of care. Even absence—empty space, muted sound, closed doors—takes on meaning. These elements shape how families gather, how staff move, and how memory takes root.

The chapters that follow move through the life cycle of a hospice room, from arrival to vigil, from death to renewal. They examine how ritual, culture, sound, light, and movement interact with human vulnerability. The intent is not to romanticize dying but, rather, to honor it as a deeply human experience that deserves thoughtfulness, humility, and care.

This work is grounded in lived experience. The observations within these pages emerge from repeated encounters with families navigating uncertainty, reconciliation, love, and grief. They reflect patterns seen over time rather than isolated moments. Although the language may feel contemplative, the insights are practical, shaped by what consistently eases distress and what quietly amplifies it.

Importantly, this book centers flexibility. Families arrive carrying histories, beliefs, conflicts, and hopes that cannot be predicted or neatly categorized. Spaces that honor this complexity do not impose meaning; they allow meaning to emerge. Design, in this context, becomes an act of listening rather than control.

Caregivers, too, are part of the room's story. Their movements, pauses, and gestures are influenced by space as much as training. A well-designed room supports not only families but also the staff who return to it again and again, carrying cumulative emotional weight. Architecture that acknowledges this shared humanity sustains compassion rather than depleting it.

This book does not seek to define what a "good death" looks like. Such definitions are personal and varied. Instead, it asks how environments can remain open enough to hold whatever unfolds—peace or turmoil, silence or song, reconciliation or unresolved grief—without judgment or intrusion.

Quiet rooms are not empty spaces waiting to be filled. They are vessels shaped by intention, history, and care. They remember. They teach. They offer continuity even as lives end within them.

If this book succeeds, it will do so quietly. It will encourage readers—designers, clinicians, administrators, and caregivers—to pause, notice, and consider how space participates in moments that matter most. It will suggest that compassion can be built, not only practiced.

Ultimately, this work is an invitation: to slow down, to observe more carefully, and to recognize that even at the end of life, the environment can affirm dignity, presence, and belonging.

Before entering the chapters that follow, take a moment. Breathe. Notice the room around you. The work begins there.

Acknowledgments

This book exists because of people who showed me, often without realizing it, how to sit with complexity, uncertainty, and human vulnerability. Some taught through instruction, others through example, and many simply by being present when presence was hardest to sustain.

First, to my wife, Dana—thank you for the patience that rarely gets named and the steadiness that makes long work possible. This book was shaped in quiet hours, in moments taken from shared time, and in emotional spaces that do not always leave visible marks. Your support was not loud, but it was constant. That constancy made everything else achievable.

To Penney, my first hospice administrator, I owe a debt that extends beyond professional guidance. You modeled leadership rooted in integrity, discernment, and humanity long before those words became fashionable. You trusted clinical intuition, respected the emotional labor of hospice work, and insisted that dignity mattered—not just for patients, but for staff as well. Much of what appears in these pages traces back to lessons learned under your leadership, whether directly spoken or quietly demonstrated.

I am grateful to the colleagues I worked beside—nurses, aides, social workers, chaplains, physicians, volunteers, and support staff—who carried the weight of this work day after day. Your willingness to show up fully, even when exhausted, shaped my understanding of care more than any textbook ever could. The rooms described in this book were never held by architecture alone; they were held by you.

To the families who allowed me into their most fragile moments: Thank you for your trust. You shared stories, silences, anger, tenderness, and love without knowing how deeply those moments would echo. Although details have been altered and identities protected, the truths remain intact. This book is, in many ways, a reflection of what you taught me about courage, grief, and presence.

I also acknowledge the patients whose lives intersected with mine at the end of their journeys. Even when words were no longer possible, meaning was communicated through gesture, breath, and stillness. These encounters reshaped my understanding of what it means to witness, rather than fix, and to honor rather than intervene.

To my family and friends who supported this work from a distance—through encouragement, patience, and quiet understanding—thank you for allowing me the space to carry stories that could not always be shared at the dinner table. Your steadiness mattered more than you may realize.

This book was not written to offer conclusions but, rather, to invite attention. It stands on the shoulders of countless unseen moments, ordinary acts of care, and rooms that held more than they were ever designed to hold. To all who contributed to those moments—named and unnamed—this work belongs to you as much as it does to me.

Finally, to those who will carry this work forward—caregivers, designers, administrators, and readers—may you continue to notice what is often overlooked. May you trust the power of presence. And may the spaces you shape, in whatever way you shape them, hold people gently when it matters most.

Prologue

There is a moment, unmistakable yet impossible to prepare for, when someone steps into a hospice room for the first time and the familiar world—the pace, the demands, the noise—slips away behind them like a coat shrugged off at the door. The hallway may have been full of chatter, rolling carts, or hurried footsteps, but the threshold to the room breaks that momentum. Crossing into a hospice room feels like entering a different physics of time, a pocket of stillness carved with intention. The door doesn't simply swing open; it reveals a space where everything slows, where the ceiling feels taller and the air feels gentler, where quiet is not the absence of sound but the presence of care.

For families arriving shaken by prognosis or worn thin by months of vigil at home, the room offers an immediate exhale. Light settles in pools instead of glare, illuminating the space with a warmth that calms rather than commands. The furniture is arranged with a deliberate softness—balanced, uncluttered, reassuring. The air carries a subtle scent of clean linens, warm towels, or perhaps lavender from a recent comfort bath. Nothing in the space overwhelms; instead, it wraps around the visitor like a soft shawl, inviting them to let their shoulders lower, their breath deepen, and their fear ebb just a little.

Every hospice room holds a dual identity: part sanctuary, part home. Families enter carrying the ordinary clutter of daily life—snacks in plastic bags, blankets folded hurriedly from the couch, a laptop still buzzing with unanswered emails. These items, chaotic as they are, begin to settle into the architecture of the room. A scarf draped over a chair becomes a sign of a daughter standing vigil. A favorite mug placed near the sink becomes a morning ritual of grounding. A half-read paperback resting on the bedside table becomes a quiet promise not to leave. Slowly, gently, the room absorbs these objects and gives them new emotional weight.

The patient shapes the room even more. No two lives imprint the space in the same way. Some patients bring a brightness that catches in the window glass and lingers in the air long after laughter fades. Others bring a depth of stillness that makes even the smallest sound—the turning of a page, the brush of fabric, a whisper—feel sacred. Some arrive surrounded by decades of memories, photos lining the shelves and voices filling every corner. Others arrive alone or nearly so, and the room offers companionship without judgment, its quiet holding their solitude with dignity rather than emptiness. The architecture adapts, almost intuitively, to what the person needs most.

At the center of the room, the bed becomes the heart of the space. It is never simply furniture—it is the axis of care, the hearth of the final chapter, the place where breath becomes ritual and touch becomes legacy. Nurses move around it with a practiced grace, smoothing covers, positioning pillows, offering warm cloths in gestures that feel both professional and profoundly tender. The placement of the bed—angled toward the window, set back from the door—signals something essential: *This is a place where a human life is ending, and it will be tended with gentleness.*

The window becomes a companion in these final days. Through it, the outside world continues in soft, steady rhythms—leaves shifting in the wind, birds hopping between branches, clouds drifting across blue or gray sky. Sometimes the sun casts golden light across the linens; other times rain runs in streaks down the glass like a quiet lament. At night, moonlight settles in a thin, silvery layer at the edge of the bed, creating pathways of calm that seem almost otherworldly. Families sit beside the window, watching the world move gently around their grief, finding comfort in the constancy of nature.

Light shapes the emotional climate of the room more than anything else. Nurses dim the lamps with deliberate care, signaling transitions without speaking a word. Daylight softens as it moves across the walls, creating slow shifts that help anchor restless minds. In the evening, small pockets of light form islands of intimacy around the bed, encouraging families to lean closer, to hold hands, to share stories. Night is not darkness here; it is a softer version of day, a quiet canvas for reflection, hope, or simply presence. The dance between shadow and glow becomes its own ritual.

The chair by the window becomes the vigil seat. Across hours or days or weeks, it holds the weight of devotion—spouses curling into its corners, children spinning between wakefulness and sleep, old friends sitting silently with hands folded in their laps. The chair becomes an anchor for those who cannot control the ending but can choose to stay near it. Sometimes, when the room is emptied after a passing, someone will pause and touch the back of this chair as if acknowledging its role as witness. In its fabric, its creases, its worn armrests, a story has been told.

On the bedside table, objects gather like small constellations of meaning. A framed wedding photo softened at the edges from decades of dusting. A child's drawing. A worn prayer book. A rosary polished by years of touch. A hairbrush, a tube of lip balm, a single blooming flower in a cup. Ordinary items—humble, unremarkable—become the vessels through which love continues to be expressed. The hospice room turns these objects into symbolic anchors, each one holding a piece of the person's story, each one offering something to hold onto as the letting-go draws near.

In the corners of the room, time moves differently. Hours stretch and contract in unpredictable patterns, as though the room operates on a clock entirely separate from the rest of the world. Families lose track of whether it is morning or evening, whether minutes or hours have passed since the last breath shift or whispered conversation. The architecture does not fight this altered state—it embraces it. Soft lighting, quiet hallways, and the absence of harsh institutional cues allow time to dissolve gently, reducing the frantic push of the outside world.

Ritual begins to shape the space, often without anyone naming it as such. A daughter wipes her mother's forehead each morning with a warm cloth. A husband reads one poem every night from a favorite book. A son gently adjusts his father's blanket each time it slips. Nurses too engage in rituals of care, smoothing linens with slow hands, dimming lights in a sequence as familiar as prayer, pausing at the doorway after each visit to offer a silent wish for comfort. These rituals give the room a rhythm, a heartbeat, a sense of continuity even as life wanes.

Sometimes, the room fills with stories—told aloud, whispered through tears, or spoken directly to the patient even after responsiveness fades. These stories settle into the walls, becoming part of the emotional architecture. The room absorbs them without judgment: the triumphs, the failures, the regrets, the laughter, the memories of childhood summers or long marriages or small, perfect moments that defined a life. The physical space becomes a quiet witness, holding these stories as gently as it holds the person who is leaving.

And sometimes, there is no story spoken aloud at all. Instead, the room holds silence—long stretches of it—broken only by the soft hum of the oxygen machine or the sound of shifting fabric. In these moments, silence becomes its own language, saying what cannot be said, revealing what cannot be articulated. The quiet room honors both forms of expression, welcoming words and wordlessness with equal compassion.

As the final hours approach, the room often grows even quieter. Families speak in murmurs. Nurses move with increased softness. Light dims slowly, settling into a warm glow near the bed. Breath becomes the central sound, rising and falling like a tide. In this suspended time, the room feels like a vessel—steady, warm, protective—carrying everyone within it through the final stretch of a long journey.

When the moment of passing arrives, it often does so gently. A nurse may place a hand over the patient's heart or hold their hand for a final moment. A family member may lean in to whisper a last goodbye. Sometimes there is a final exhale that seems to echo through the room. Sometimes the transition is so quiet it is noticed only when someone looks at the stillness and understands. In this moment, the room shifts again, becoming a space of tenderness, of reverence, of deep exhale.

Afterward, the rituals continue. A nurse may dim the light further. A spouse might rest their forehead on the bedrail. A child may touch the patient's hand one last time. The window might catch a shift in wind or light that feels, to those who remain, like some small acknowledgment of passage. The room holds these moments with infinite patience.

In the minutes or hours following a death, the room becomes a sanctuary for grief. Families linger, sometimes in silence, sometimes sharing memories, sometimes simply holding each other as though trying to anchor themselves in a new and unfamiliar world. The architecture does not rush them. The design does not intrude. The room offers its quiet as a form of comfort, asking nothing in return.

When the family finally leaves, the room enters a different kind of quiet—one marked not by vigil but by completion. Nurses perform the room-reset ritual with reverence: smoothing the sheets, folding blankets, adjusting the lamp, arranging furniture with gentle hands. In these gestures lives an acknowledgment that this space has hosted something sacred, that the walls have borne witness to a final chapter deserving of honor.

And then, eventually, the door will reopen for another family, another patient, another story. The room will shift again, responding to the needs of those who enter, reshaping itself around new grief, new love, new rituals, new breaths. It will do so with the same quiet, humble dignity it has offered countless times before.

This is the essence of the quiet room—a place built not merely to house the end of life, but to honor it. A place where architecture becomes an act of compassion, where objects become anchors of presence, where light becomes a form of care. A place where dying is not an abandonment but a vigil, not an emergency but a sacred transition. A place where the final pages of a life are written in gentleness, witness, and profound quiet.

And it is here, in this room where the world slows and the heart listens differently, that the story of designing compassion truly begins.

1

The Architecture of Stillness

The experience of quiet inside a hospice room does not simply arise from the absence of noise. It is produced—carefully, deliberately—through the materials, geometry, textures, and sensory choreography that surround the patient and family. Architects often speak of "atmosphere," a term that sounds ephemeral but is shaped by dozens of micro-decisions: how softly a door closes, how the floor absorbs sound, how the lighting diffuses rather than pierces. In hospice, quiet is not a luxury—it is a form of care. The room must feel like a gentler world nested inside a louder one, a space where emotional burden can soften just enough for families to breathe again.

Creating that kind of quiet begins with the walls. In many modern hospices, walls are lined with sound-absorbing panels disguised as art, woven textiles, or warm neutral surfaces that read as home rather than institution. Acoustic tiles overhead dampen footsteps in the hallway. Even the internal structure—cork backing beneath drywall, insulation placed with precision—plays a role in reducing the hard echoes that make hospital spaces feel cold. When a nurse pulls a chair across the floor or when a visitor gently sets down a cup of water, the sound is subdued, softened, absorbed by the space rather than amplified. This is architectural empathy expressed through materials.

The door becomes another vital instrument of quiet. In traditional medical settings, doors slam, click, or rattle, each sound a sharp reminder of vulnerability. In a hospice room, soft-closing hinges and silicone-edged seals reduce abrupt noise. The door glides rather than shuts, creating a transition that feels respectful rather than intrusive. Families often describe this as one of the first indicators that the room is different from a hospital—a sense that the space honors the human experience unfolding inside. The door becomes a boundary not only of privacy but also of peace, marking the room as a refuge where noise has been intentionally tamed.

Clutter-free sightlines play a subtler but equally important role in emotional ease. When a patient lies in bed and looks toward the doorway or window, the geometry of the room should feel predictable and calm. Clean lines, minimal protrusions, and gently curved transitions create a visual field that does not demand cognitive processing. A cluttered or chaotic visual environment can increase agitation, especially for patients with delirium or sensory sensitivity. Simplified spatial geometry reduces the number of decisions the brain must make, allowing patients—many of whom are already fatigued—to relax into the environment without subconscious effort.

Researchers in environmental psychology have long noted the connection between spatial clarity and emotional regulation, even in nonmedical settings. Visual confusion, such as too many intersecting lines, unpredictable corners, or asymmetrical door placements, can activate subtle fight-or-flight responses, especially when someone is already vulnerable or disoriented. In hospice care, where patients may slip in and out of wakefulness, clarity of space becomes more than aesthetics—it becomes mental comfort.[1] The geometry tells the body, *You are safe. Nothing here will surprise you.*

This design clarity applies not only to walls and doors but also to furniture placement. A single armchair positioned at an angle rather than jutting into the pathway can change the entire emotional reading of the room. Tables with rounded corners, beds placed so the view opens outward rather than crowding into a wall, and storage spaces recessed rather than protruding all contribute to an environment in which movement feels natural and unobstructed. Families may not consciously notice these choices, but their bodies respond nonetheless, relaxing shoulders, slowing breaths, allowing grief to unfold without the interference of environmental stress.

Another component of emotional ease is what architects call "legible circulation"—the intuitive sense of how to move through space. In a hospice room, this means the bathroom is easy to locate without confusion, the nurse can enter without startling the patient, and family members can find a comfortable place to sit without feeling like they are intruding on medical equipment. The room must be arranged so that even someone visiting for the first time understands instantly how to inhabit it. Predictability, at the end of life, becomes a source of immense psychological comfort.

Nighttime presents its own set of design challenges. Patients often experience heightened fear, restlessness, or hallucinations after dark, especially when nearing the end of life. Soft night lighting—indirect light-emitting diodes (LEDs) positioned along floor trim or behind headboards—provides gentle orientation without overwhelming the senses. Harsh overhead lights can cause panic or confusion; even the sound of a fluorescent fixture buzzing can fray the nerves of a patient already struggling with anxiety or delirium. Low, warm lighting supports circadian rhythm, reduces the risk of nighttime agitation, and helps family members navigate the space without disrupting the patient's sleep.

Sensory load reduction goes beyond light and sound. It includes textures, scents, and even air movement. A hospice room avoids strong chemical odors in favor of subtle natural scents: fresh linens, soft wood, occasionally a hint of lavender from a diffuser used sparingly. Fabrics are chosen not only for durability but also for sensory comfort—cotton, linen blends, and soft upholstery that invites touch. The heating, ventilation, and air conditioning system is calibrated to avoid harsh airflow directly onto the patient, providing ventilation without discomfort. All of these choices weave together to create a sensory environment that gently lowers the body's stress responses.

In traditional hospital rooms, medical equipment often dominates the visual field: blinking monitors, sharp metal edges, coiled wires. Hospice design deliberately conceals or softens these elements. Oxygen tubing can be hidden within built-in channels. Storage cabinets close smoothly to obscure supplies. Syringe pumps fit into recessed spaces. Even the trash and linen bins are often concealed behind wood panels that blend with the rest of the room. This concealment is not cosmetic vanity—it is a psychological intervention. For patients and families, the fewer reminders of medical struggle, the more space remains for emotional presence.

The concept of "emotional predictability" is especially powerful in the final weeks of life. Patients may drift through states of confusion, lucidity, fear, and peace, sometimes within hours. A room with no sudden corners, no bright unexpected glare, and no disorienting layout becomes an anchor. The stability of the environment offers grounding when the internal world feels unstable. Even the rhythm of how shadows fall at different times of day can contribute to a sense of continuity that counterbalances the patient's shifting consciousness.

One of the most compelling illustrations of how design affects emotional ease comes from comparing traditional hospital rooms with hospice rooms created with soft movement in mind. In a typical hospital setting, a patient lying in bed often sees stark white walls, exposed pipes, and the harsh geometry of metal bed rails. The hallway beyond the door is a flurry of voices, rolling carts, and mechanical noise. The body remains on alert, as if bracing for interruption. By contrast, a hospice room offers a gentle visual field: warm hues, filtered natural light, soft surfaces, and slowed visual rhythm. The difference is immediate and profound—families report feeling calmer the moment they enter.[2]

Consider the movement of staff within the room. In a standard hospital space, the layout forces nurses to maneuver awkwardly around equipment, creating accidental noise or abrupt movement. In a hospice room designed for quiet, pathways are wide and unobstructed, allowing staff to glide rather than scramble. A nurse can approach the patient from the side rather than looming over them. Linens can be changed without jarring the furniture. These small movements accumulate into an atmosphere of smoothness, a choreography of care that patients perceive even when sedated or semiconscious.

Emotional ease is also shaped by the room's relationship to nature. Even if the view is modest—a courtyard, a tree, a strip of sky—the presence of the natural world reinforces calm. The window becomes a steady companion, offering visual continuity even when time becomes disjointed. Studies show that exposure to natural light and outdoor views reduces anxiety and improves emotional stability for patients nearing end of life.[3] In hospice architecture, the window is not merely a feature—it is a lifeline to the rhythms of the world.

The palette of colors in a hospice room further shapes the emotional experience. Soft earth tones, muted greens, gentle creams, and warm wood create a backdrop that soothes rather than stimulates. These colors absorb light rather than reflecting it harshly, contributing to the room's overall sense of quiet. Color psychology suggests that muted palettes can reduce cortisol levels and support emotional regulation, especially in high-stress environments. In hospice, color becomes a silent partner in care.

Furniture selection also supports emotional predictability. Chairs are upholstered in fabrics that read as residential rather than clinical; tables are placed thoughtfully so families can reach them without disturbing the patient. The bed, although medically functional, is designed to look less like a machine and more like a place of rest. This blending of residential comfort with medical necessity transforms the room into an environment in which families feel permitted to relax, cry, laugh, or simply be present without feeling as though they are intruding on a sterile workspace.

One of the profound truths of hospice care is that the room becomes a container for emotion. Families bring their fear, their hope, their memories, their uncertainty. The environment must absorb these emotions without amplifying them. A quiet room allows grief to settle gently rather than crash; it gives families space to speak to one another in tones that feel natural. The architecture becomes a participant in the emotional process, shaping not only the experience of dying but also the experience of loving someone through their dying.

Material choice reinforces dignity—a concept often overlooked in medical architecture. The feel of a wooden handrail instead of cold metal, the softness of a blanket, and the warmth of a lamp instead of fluorescent glare all convey respect for the patient's humanity. These are not trivial features—they are signals of compassion embedded in the built environment. In moments when families feel powerless, these small dignities offer comfort.

Even the acoustics of footsteps matter. In a hospice room, flooring is chosen to minimize sound: cushioned vinyl, cork composites, or wood-textured laminate that absorbs rather than echoes. The soft thud of a nurse entering the room becomes a kind of reassurance rather than a disruption. Families often report that they begin to recognize staff members by the rhythm of their footsteps, each pattern forming part of the room's auditory landscape—a quiet symphony of care.

The emotional impact of such an environment cannot be overstated. When patients feel calmer, their breathing slows, anxiety diminishes, and rest becomes more accessible. Families feel safer expressing their emotions openly.

Conversations flow more naturally. The room becomes a shared sanctuary rather than a battlefield. In this way, architectural quiet becomes a form of medicine—nonpharmacological yet profoundly therapeutic.

Ultimately, designing for emotional ease is an act of profound compassion. It acknowledges that dying is not only a medical event but also a deeply human one, filled with vulnerability and meaning. The hospice room is designed not to fix or cure but to cradle—to hold the emotional weight of a family's final chapter with gentleness, dignity, and clarity. Within its walls, architecture becomes more than structure; it becomes a companion to the dying and a witness to love.

The first impression upon entering a hospice room is often subconscious, yet it sets the tone for every interaction within. Beyond light, color, and sound, the proportions and spatial layout shape the emotional experience profoundly. Ceiling height, room width, the distance between furniture, and the arrangement of visual elements all communicate subtle psychological cues. Patients who enter spaces with low ceilings or compressed layouts frequently report feelings of unease or even claustrophobia. Conversely, ceilings that rise just enough above the eye line can create an expansive feeling, a subtle sense of openness that resonates with the spiritual dimension of end-of-life care.[4]

Ceiling height interacts not only with psychological perception but also with acoustics and light. Higher ceilings allow sound to disperse rather than bounce sharply, reducing echoes that might make the space feel tense. Daylight entering from upper level windows spreads more evenly, softening shadows and creating a gentle visual gradient. Patients often describe this as a "breathing space," a room that feels less confining and more capable of holding both stillness and emotion. This interplay of height, light, and air contributes to a perception of spaciousness that is more than physical—it is emotional, almost sacred in quality.

One subtle but powerful design principle concerns the visibility of the patient bed. In conventional hospital settings, the bed is often the first object in view upon entry, emphasizing illness, vulnerability, and clinical attention. In a hospice room, this approach is intentionally reversed. The bed should never dominate the threshold view; instead, the first impression might be a chair by the window, a low table with personal items, or an unobstructed visual corridor toward natural light. This spatial decision preserves dignity, allowing families and patients to experience the room as a sanctuary rather than a medical tableau. It reinforces the idea that the room supports life and presence, not just the clinical act of dying.

Within the room, architects and designers use the concept of "micro-zones" to create functional and emotional compartments. The vigil zone encompasses the bedside, where patients spend most of their time and where family and staff provide direct care. The bed remains central here, but surrounding furniture, lighting, and surfaces are deliberately arranged to allow unobstructed movement and intimate engagement. Chairs, side tables, and low shelves are positioned to support extended presence, allowing hands to be held, blankets to be adjusted, or soft words whispered without interference.

The reflection zone is typically defined by the window chair or a small alcove bathed in natural light. This zone allows patients and families moments of mental and emotional respite. It may accommodate quiet reading, meditation, journaling, or silent observation of the external environment. The reflection zone is intentionally separated from the vigil zone to give a sense of choice: Patients or family members can move physically and psychologically within the room according to their needs.

The staff zone is a clinical alcove designed to allow unobtrusive delivery of care. Nurses and aides need access to medication, supplies, and monitoring equipment without interrupting the patient's experience or intruding upon family interactions. Thoughtful placement of cabinets, drawers, and medical devices reduces cross-room travel, minimizes noise, and prevents inadvertent exposure of equipment that might otherwise feel intimidating. This choreography of movement within the room becomes a form of silent communication: Staff are present but not disruptive, attending yet discreet.

Finally, the memory zone is often a small table, shelf, or alcove for personal items: photographs, cards, a journal, small mementos, or religious objects. It exists to honor presence, legacy, and personal history. Families intuitively understand the function of this zone, and patients frequently interact with it, even subtly. The memory zone allows the room to carry layered meaning: It is not only functional but also symbolic, a container for love, attention, and remembrance.

Spatial proportions are critical in defining these zones. Hallways, doorways, and walking paths must accommodate multiple users, including family members, medical staff, and mobility aids. A path that forces constant sidestepping or blocking creates stress; generous widths, gentle curves, and smooth transitions allow the room to function as a coordinated choreography of care. Every element—wall, chair, table, curtain—plays a role in orchestrating movement so that the act of caregiving feels effortless rather than obstructed.

Even the placement of electrical outlets and medical connections is part of spatial breathing. Outlets that are too low or positioned awkwardly create unnecessary stooping or twisting, breaking the flow of movement. Thoughtful positioning reduces the number of times staff must cross the room to retrieve or adjust equipment, which preserves both the patient's sense of calm and the family's experience of dignity. In this sense, efficiency and emotional ease are inseparable: The less friction in staff movement, the less intrusion into the sanctuary of the room.

Architects often use proportion to influence psychological perception. A room with a low, narrow ceiling can subconsciously compress the mind, creating tension, whereas a modestly higher ceiling with gentle horizontal lines fosters expansiveness without emptiness. Furniture height, window sill placement, and counter levels are similarly calibrated to maintain sightlines that feel balanced. Patients in such spaces report feeling less confined and more able to orient themselves independently.

Sightlines also influence how families perceive the flow of the room. When each micro-zone is intuitively legible, visitors quickly understand where to sit, where to stand, and how to move without hesitation. Families often report an immediate sense of coherence, noting that they "just know" how to inhabit the room. This clarity reduces anxiety, allowing emotional energy to focus on presence rather than navigation. The room's structure communicates care silently and constantly.

The relationship between zones is fluid, not rigid. A family member may occupy the reflection zone at one moment and then move to the vigil zone to offer touch or words of comfort. The patient may drift from bed to window chair if mobility permits, guided by light, view, or personal ritual. The flow between zones is reinforced by materials and textures: Soft rugs or gentle transitions between flooring types subtly cue movement, while continuous wall colors or patterns unify the space visually.

Ceiling height, again, plays a role in this choreography. Slightly higher ceilings over the vigil zone can create a sense of openness around the bed, reducing feelings of confinement, while lower ceilings in the staff zone or alcove can make clinical equipment feel integrated rather than imposing. This variation in vertical space adds subtle cues that guide attention, comfort, and function without overt signage.

Natural light serves as a key navigational and emotional guide within microzones. The reflection zone typically receives the most daylight, offering a visual destination. Shadows and light gradients subtly demarcate areas, helping patients and families intuitively understand spatial hierarchy. Lighting also reinforces temporal orientation—morning, afternoon, and evening light cues assist with circadian rhythm, supporting emotional and physiological regulation.

Flow extends to furniture arrangement. Chairs are positioned to encourage eye contact, but not to dominate space. Tables for memory items are accessible yet unobtrusive. Beds are centered within the vigil zone but not aligned directly with the door, preserving dignity and privacy. The cumulative effect is an environment that feels purposeful and predictable, reducing cognitive load and reinforcing a sense of control during a vulnerable time.

The choreography of staff movement is especially important in larger hospice rooms or suites. By carefully mapping how nurses, aides, and volunteers access equipment, designers minimize accidental collisions, disruptive foot traffic, or noise intrusion. This allows care to unfold as a seamless dance, where every gesture is intentional and every pause respectful. Families perceive this flow subconsciously: The room "feels right," a combination of movement, sightlines, and proportionality.

Spatial breathing also considers the psychological impact of thresholds and entry points. A visitor's approach to the room should be gradual, providing a sense of arrival and transition from the outside world. Doorways are sized to accommodate multiple people, including those with mobility devices, without creating bottlenecks. Hallway-to-room transitions may include slight lighting adjustments, textured flooring, or gentle visual cues that signal the change from public to private, from ordinary to sanctuary.

The room's flow must support emotional and relational dynamics. Zones allow multiple family members to gather without crowding, to sit quietly, or to engage in caregiving rituals without interfering with one another. Staff can enter and exit unobtrusively, attending to clinical needs while respecting intimacy. The spatial orchestration fosters harmony, reducing tension and supporting a calm, dignified environment for the patient's final days.

Finally, the patient's perception of spatial coherence reinforces agency and orientation. A room with clearly defined zones, intuitive circulation, and proportional balance reduces fear and disorientation. Patients report feeling "in command" simply by knowing where to rest, where to see the sky, or where family members might gather. The architecture itself becomes a nonverbal form of guidance, offering reassurance and continuity even when verbal communication is limited.

The hospice room threshold is more than a structural necessity—it is the portal between the world outside and the intimate universe within. A visitor's first encounter with the room shapes emotional response, whether consciously or subliminally. A widened, unobstructed doorway communicates openness, safety, and welcome. Unlike the narrow, clinical entrances of traditional hospitals, a hospice threshold signals that this is a space deliberately designed to hold life, memory, and presence, even as the patient nears its end.[5]

Unobstructed thresholds also serve a symbolic function, marking a transition from ordinary time to the "sacred time" of hospice. Patients and families crossing this boundary may not verbalize the change, yet the body and mind respond to the subtle cues embedded in architectural design. The width of the door, the absence of visual clutter in the entryway, and the smoothness of movement across the threshold reduce the anticipatory tension that often accompanies hospital visits. Here, the act of entering becomes a ritual of acknowledgment and care.

The "first view" into the room profoundly impacts emotional response. When the patient bed is the first object visible, it may evoke anxiety or a sense of vulnerability. In contrast, arranging the room so that light, nature, or artwork greets the eye creates a gentle welcome. A window framed with soft curtains, a small piece of serene art, or even a view of a tree in a courtyard becomes a conscious visual cue that the room is a sanctuary. The first glimpse is an emotional primer, shaping how visitors and family members experience the room before they even reach the bedside.[6]

The entrance is more than visual—it is tactile and auditory. Door materials, handle textures, and the sound of closure play a role in sustaining or disrupting quiet. A hollow door with a metallic latch that clicks sharply can fracture the fragile calm of the room. Conversely, a solid wood or composite door with a soft-close mechanism conveys stability, dignity, and respect. Even subtle tactile choices, such as a smooth handle that feels natural in the hand, contribute to a sense of welcome and care. These design elements, although often unnoticed, have cumulative psychological weight.

Lighting at the doorway also warrants meticulous consideration. Soft, indirect illumination reduces the cognitive and emotional shock of transition. When a family member enters from a bright hallway into a room with gentle ambient light, their eyes adjust gradually, and their nervous system responds with relief rather than tension. Lighting can be layered: Low-level sconces, concealed LED strips, or diffused natural light create a gradient of brightness that signals calm. Threshold lighting functions almost like a verbal cue: *This is a place for peace.*

Thresholds carry cultural significance, too. Across societies, entrances are imbued with meaning in end-of-life rituals. In many Eastern traditions, entering a room in which someone is dying is an act of reverence; thresholds are often cleared, adorned, or prepared to mark the transition from ordinary life to sacred passage. In Western hospice practice, subtle architectural gestures—widened doors, clear sightlines, and smooth transitions—echo this cultural intuition, even without explicit ritual. The threshold becomes a liminal space, a physical manifestation of the psychological and spiritual passage taking place.

The width and materiality of doors are also critical for accessibility. Wheelchairs, walkers, and gurneys must pass without obstruction, yet functional necessity does not preclude aesthetic and emotional design. Wider doors allow the patient to remain central to the room's composition, maintaining dignity while accommodating the practical realities of care. Threshold design is thus an intersection of function, symbolism, and emotional resonance.

Even the visual treatment of door frames and surrounding walls affects perception. Minimal trim, subtle color contrasts, and the avoidance of harsh edges prevent the doorway from feeling like a barrier. Softly curved frames or muted tones create a sense of continuity between the hallway and the room itself. Families often remark, even subconsciously, on the difference: The entry feels "gentle," setting the stage for a calm and composed encounter with the patient.

The concept of "first glimpse" extends beyond what is immediately visible. Designers often create layered sightlines so that upon entering, the eye encounters depth and complexity without confusion. A distant window, a framed piece of artwork, or a subtle architectural detail beyond the doorway provides an anchor for attention, guiding the visitor naturally toward areas of significance, such as the reflection and memory zones. These visual cues reduce the cognitive load associated with unfamiliar space, promoting comfort and orientation.

Auditory considerations at the threshold are equally crucial. Hallway noise, intercoms, or rolling carts can intrude abruptly if the doorway does not buffer sound. Acoustic materials within the door and surrounding walls prevent sudden noise from breaking the calm. Even the small sound of the door closing must be considered: A soft, weighted mechanism avoids an abrupt interruption of quiet, preserving the emotional atmosphere the patient and family require.

The threshold also subtly regulates the psychological pacing of entrance. Entering too abruptly, especially in multi-family or multi-staff visits, can overwhelm both patient and loved ones. Wider doors and unobstructed sightlines allow a gradual arrival, a slow unfolding into the room. Families can pause, orient themselves, and adjust their pace of approach. The doorway itself becomes a silent facilitator of composure, shaping the rhythm of human presence.

Threshold design interacts with cultural and spiritual sensibilities. In some traditions, approaching a dying person requires steps of purification, attention, or blessing. Even in secular hospices, creating an unobtrusive but ceremonious approach honors the inherent gravity of the moment. Architectural gestures—subtle elevation changes, visual markers, or directional lighting—function as nonverbal acknowledgment that the room is distinct from the everyday world, a site for care, memory, and final presence.

The visual field immediately beyond the doorway should minimize clinical cues. Equipment, monitors, and other medical apparatus are concealed behind panels or positioned out of the first line of sight. This strategy allows families to encounter the human and personal aspects of the room first, softening the emotional impact of medical necessity. The room's design thus prioritizes the psychological well-being of those entering, emphasizing presence and dignity over clinical function.

The use of natural light or art at the threshold is more than aesthetic—it is emotionally stabilizing. Light carries directional information, creates mood, and subtly communicates safety. A small artwork or view of a tree beyond the doorway functions as a psychological anchor, drawing attention outward, providing respite for the mind, and offering continuity between interior space and the broader world. These visual and environmental cues shape experience before words are spoken.

Door hardware becomes part of the threshold experience. Handles should operate smoothly, without abrupt resistance or vibration, signaling that the room is responsive and accommodating. Materials that convey warmth, such as brushed metals or wood composites, reinforce tactile comfort. The absence of industrial coldness in the threshold communicates care and intentionality, even before the visitor reaches the patient.

The threshold is not static—it must accommodate the dynamic flow of people and movement. Staff entering for medication or observation, family members arriving together, and volunteers bringing comfort items all must pass without interfering with one another or the patient. Thoughtful proportioning and visual transparency prevent collisions, reduce accidental noise, and maintain the room's calm, reinforcing the choreography of hospice care.

Soft, indirect lighting at the threshold also aids orientation. Light can subtly mark the transition between hallway and sanctuary, helping patients recognize the room as a distinct space. Gradual light gradients prevent sensory shock and support both physical and emotional comfort. Families may unconsciously respond to this lighting, their stress levels lowering as they enter, allowing attention to shift naturally to the patient rather than the environment.

The material and acoustic treatment of the threshold, combined with sightlines and lighting, collectively influence emotional perception. Patients frequently respond positively to entrances that feel spacious, quiet, and visually coherent. Even small improvements—such as a door that closes without a bang, a window visible from the entry, or a soft glow illuminating a corridor—reinforce the overall experience of calm, thus reinforcing the sanctuary-like quality of the hospice room.

Threshold design also functions as a micro-orientation tool. Families intuitively grasp room zones—reflection, vigil, memory, and staff—once the doorway provides a coherent point of entry. Clear sightlines, light gradients, and unobstructed access allow newcomers to understand where to sit, where to approach the bedside, and where objects of personal meaning are placed. The spatial logic established at the threshold resonates throughout the visit, shaping comfort, interaction, and presence.

Finally, thresholds remind us that hospice care is a collaborative act between architecture, caregiving, and human perception. Every choice—from door width to closure sound, from lighting gradient to sightline—interacts with emotion, cognition, and ritual. The first glimpse is not a trivial design decision; it is the initial gesture of compassion, setting the stage for the patient, family, and staff to inhabit the space together in dignity, presence, and profound stillness.

The choice of materials within a hospice room is far more than aesthetic—it is an extension of care, a tactile and visual language that communicates calm, safety, and dignity. Each surface, each texture, has the potential to soothe or to provoke unease. From the first moment a hand brushes a table to the subtle reflection of light off a wall, materials anchor the emotional and sensory experience.

Designers speak of a "taxonomy of calm"—a careful selection of elements that, collectively, form a coherent, reassuring environment.

Natural woods such as birch, maple, and walnut are central to this taxonomy. Their soft grains, matte finishes, and warm color tones convey a sense of life and continuity. Birch, for example, presents subtle variegation that is never repetitive, offering visual interest without overstimulation. Wood surfaces reduce the sharpness of light reflections, create soft acoustic absorption, and provide warmth under the hand. The familiarity of wood evokes domesticity and comfort, bridging the gap between clinical care and homelike intimacy.

Matte textures extend this principle into other surfaces: Walls, cabinetry, and decorative panels benefit from finishes that scatter light gently rather than bouncing it harshly. Matte plaster, soft-painted walls, or textured wallpaper reduce glare and visual fatigue, supporting emotional ease. Patients with fragile vision, sensitivity to light, or cognitive vulnerability respond positively to the subtle diffusion, finding the environment easier to inhabit without conscious effort.

Textiles, too, play a crucial role in tactile psychology. Linen upholstery, wool throws, cotton blankets, and even carefully woven upholstery invite touch, a reminder that the body and environment are in dialogue. These fabrics offer a sense of connection, a physical reassurance that contrasts with the sterility of purely clinical materials. By contrast, glossy plastics or cold synthetic surfaces repel touch, signaling distance and impermanence. Avoiding these materials is essential in creating a room that encourages gentle, repeated interaction with one's surroundings.

Ceramic, stone, and clay surfaces provide visual and tactile grounding. Their matte finishes, subtle textural variation, and cool but non-alien temperature create moments of sensory pause. A small ceramic vase on a shelf, a clay bowl holding mementos, or a stone window-sill can become both functional objects and anchors for attention, inviting presence rather than distraction. The subtle irregularities in these materials reinforce a sense of authenticity, countering the sterile uniformity of clinical spaces.

Temperature interacts with material in profound ways. Warm-touch materials such as wood, textiles, and soft leather feel inviting, whereas metallic or glazed surfaces feel cold, distant, or even intimidating. Patients' tactile sensitivity is often heightened near the end of life; materials that feel welcoming under the hand can provide reassurance, whereas cold surfaces reinforce separation and clinical impersonality. Designers must consider not only visual aesthetics but also the lived experience of touch, weight, and temperature in each material choice.

Patina and material aging are equally important in creating emotional resonance. Surfaces that develop subtle wear—softened edges on a wooden handrail, a slightly polished spot on a table where hands often rest—strengthen the room's "emotional archive." These traces of human presence make the space feel lived-in, safe, and familiar. Rather than appearing neglected, patina communicates care, longevity, and history, enhancing the room's role as a witness to life and memory.

Glossy floors, high-reflective plastics, and exposed stainless steel are examples of materials that evoke institutional associations. Such materials can provoke anxiety, heighten awareness of clinical authority, and reduce the perception of intimacy. Glossy surfaces exaggerate movement, increase glare, and create a sense of coldness. Minimizing these cues through matte finishes, warm tones, and softer textures transforms the room into a sanctuary rather than a facility.

Carpeting or low-pile rugs contribute additional sensory grounding. In addition to their tactile warmth underfoot, they reduce noise, muffling footsteps and incidental sounds from staff or visitors. Subtle variations in weave, color, and pattern can delineate zones—vigil, reflection, and memory—without overt barriers, reinforcing spatial understanding while maintaining calm. Even the padding beneath carpet or vinyl composite surfaces contributes to acoustic absorption, softening the room's sonic environment.

Upholstered furniture combines visual warmth with tactile comfort. Chairs and armrests must invite touch, allowing hands to rest naturally without harsh angles or unyielding surfaces. Textured linen or soft wool contrasts with smooth wood, offering multiple points of sensory engagement. This combination creates a layered, rich environment in which the body feels acknowledged and supported.

Material contrast must be subtle, deliberate, and psychologically coherent. Abrupt transitions from warm wood to cold metal or glossy plastic jar perception, even unconsciously. Smooth integration of materials—soft wood, matte paint, and natural fibers—produces visual and tactile continuity, reinforcing the room's calming effect. The interplay of textures forms a nonverbal narrative, quietly communicating care, thoughtfulness, and attention to detail.

Windowsills, counters, and small tables exemplify this principle. A windowsill in smooth, warm wood invites a hand to rest and gaze outward; a low table in soft, matte ceramic encourages placement of personal objects. These choices reflect a design philosophy that considers every interaction, intentional or incidental, as part of the patient and family experience.

Even wall finishes interact with sensory grounding. Slightly textured plaster or paint creates depth without distraction, breaking up large, featureless planes that feel institutional. Subtle gradation of color, combined with tactile interest, provides visual and psychological comfort. Patients and visitors alike respond to surfaces that communicate texture, warmth, and subtle irregularity—qualities that evoke life rather than machinery.

Light interacts with materials to enhance emotional resonance. Matte, textured surfaces diffuse and absorb light, reducing glare and creating soft shadow gradients. Natural woods and warm textiles reflect light gently, supporting circadian rhythms while reinforcing a sense of calm. The interaction of light and material produces an environment that is responsive and alive, without startling or overstimulating the senses.

Flooring surfaces must balance warmth, tactile quality, and maintenance. Wood, cork, or soft composite surfaces are preferable to cold tile or linoleum, offering both acoustic and tactile benefits. These surfaces reduce echoes, provide gentle cushioning underfoot, and maintain warmth for patients moving independently or assisted. Even subtle variations in floor texture can cue zones, supporting orientation and flow.

Door materials, handles, and wall trim contribute similarly to tactile and emotional comfort. Smooth, warm finishes and soft-closing mechanisms create reassurance, whereas hollow, metallic doors with sharp edges can signal abruptness and impersonal authority. These details, although subtle, frame the entry experience and influence ongoing perception of the room.

The layering of materials reinforces the room's emotional richness. Textiles on furniture, natural wood surfaces, ceramic or stone accents, and soft wall finishes interact to form a multisensory environment. Each layer is chosen not merely for durability or maintenance but for its capacity to invite touch, encourage presence, and ground attention in the immediate surroundings.

Maintenance and material longevity intersect with emotional considerations. Surfaces that withstand cleaning without harsh sheen or reflective distortion allow the room to remain safe, hygienic, and visually comforting. Overly glossy or industrial-clean finishes may appear antiseptic, undermining the sensory warmth required in a hospice environment. Choosing resilient, warm, and matte surfaces ensures both safety and emotional resonance.

Ultimately, materials in a hospice room are not passive; they actively participate in the care of the patient. Wood, textiles, ceramics, and stone communicate warmth, continuity, and dignity. Their tactile and visual qualities soothe, support orientation, and offer an implicit invitation to engage with the room. Through careful selection, maintenance, and layering, materials anchor emotional experience, creating an environment in which presence, memory, and comfort coexist seamlessly.

A hospice room does not exist in isolation; it functions as an ecosystem, a living container that interacts with human behavior. Architecture, materials, light, and spatial design converge to shape experience, not merely in abstract aesthetic terms but in practical, psychological, and emotional ways. The quiet room must anticipate the rhythms of daily life, the unpredictable arrival of loved ones, and the fragile trajectories of human emotion, all while maintaining a sense of dignity and calm.

At the heart of this ecosystem is the interplay between architectural stillness and human rituals. The room is designed to absorb the emotional energy of visitation, caregiving, and presence, providing boundaries that contain grief while simultaneously supporting connection. In this way, the walls, floors, and furnishings act as silent partners in care, mediating interaction and facilitating intimate moments without overt intervention.

Designing for the unpredictable is essential. Sudden visits from distant relatives, spontaneous expressions of emotion, or rapid clinical events may all occur in a single afternoon. The room must be resilient, offering zones for private reflection, family gathering, and staff care without fracturing the flow of attention or amplifying stress. Flexible seating, unobstructed pathways, and easily adjusted lighting allow the space to shift in response to these emergent needs.

End-of-life transitions, in particular, demand a room that can hold extremes of emotion. Architecture does not prevent grief, fear, or expression, but it can create a sense of containment and safety. Families report feeling "held" by a room whose dimensions, acoustics, and layout reduce visual and auditory chaos, even in moments of intense vulnerability. The room itself becomes a co-conspirator in the ritual of dying, mediating presence, attention, and care.

Spatial arrangement conveys permission for intimacy. Chairs near the bedside, a window seat for reflection, or a small alcove for private conversation signal that touch, conversation, and silent witness are not only allowed but also expected. This subtle communication is critical: In conventional clinical spaces, proximity to the patient often feels regimented or monitored. In a hospice room designed as ecosystem, architecture itself encourages closeness, supporting human relational needs without verbal explanation.

The room functions as a container for both grief and connection. Family members and caregivers often comment that even in moments of profound sadness, the space allows them to orient their attention to one another, to the patient, and to rituals that feel meaningful. Spatial coherence, soft materials, and intentional lighting reduce distraction, providing a structured emotional canvas for the delicate work of presence.

Human behavior in the room is dynamic. Visitors may move from the reflection zone to the vigil zone in response to emotional cues, often without consciously acknowledging the choreography. Architecture supports these movements: Unobstructed pathways, visual markers, and comfortable surfaces anticipate human patterns, reducing cognitive load and allowing attention to remain focused on relationships rather than navigation.

The ecosystem approach also accounts for staff behavior. Nurses, aides, and volunteers must move efficiently and quietly, delivering care while minimizing intrusion. The placement of supply alcoves, medication stations, and waste disposal allows staff to operate seamlessly, without interrupting family rituals or breaking the fragile quiet. Staff flow is choreographed alongside human interaction, forming a complex network of simultaneous activities that the room accommodates gracefully.

Objects, furnishings, and materials further reinforce the ecosystem. Chairs with soft edges and natural upholstery invite touch; low tables for mementos or ritual objects provide anchors for personal meaning; rugs and textured flooring guide movement and delineate micro-zones. The arrangement is deliberate, responding to human behavioral patterns and reinforcing an environment that is psychologically supportive and emotionally intelligent.

Thresholds and doorways play a crucial role in ecosystem dynamics. The room's entry communicates rules of engagement: The width of doors, unobstructed sightlines, and layered lighting signal that visitors may enter gently, pause, orient themselves, and adjust to the atmosphere. The threshold becomes part of the room's behavioral ecology, shaping the flow of presence and mediating first impressions.

Light within the room interacts with human activity. Adjustable natural and artificial lighting accommodates the diurnal rhythms of patients, the arrival of visitors, and the timing of spiritual or personal rituals. Soft daylight for reflection, gentle bedside illumination for evening care, and indirect accent lighting for quiet moments provide both functional visibility and emotional scaffolding for human action.

The room also responds to temporal unpredictability. Emotional intensity often fluctuates with visiting schedules, clinical events, or patient energy. Spaces designed as ecosystems accommodate these fluctuations through adaptable furnishings, mobile seating, and adjustable surfaces. Family members can cluster around the bed, spread out in the reflection zone, or withdraw into corners without architectural constraint. The environment flexes to human needs rather than imposing rigidity.

Sound management is a key component of behavioral ecology. Acoustic treatments, soft textiles, and the strategic placement of furnishings reduce auditory stress, allowing conversations, whispered prayers, or music to occur without interference. The room absorbs noise generated by movement, breathing, or emotional expression, ensuring that sound contributes to the environment without becoming overwhelming.

The patient's own behavior shapes the ecosystem. Even limited mobility influences furniture placement, spatial orientation, and interaction patterns. Designers anticipate how patients may move between the bed, chair, or window, creating corridors of flow that accommodate both physical need and emotional intent. In this sense, the room is a partner in presence: It adapts to and anticipates the human body's limitations and expressions.

The room encourages ritual without imposing it. Whether lighting a candle, reading a prayer, playing music, or simply holding a hand, these activities are supported by spatial layout, lighting, and furniture placement. Architectural design does not prescribe ritual but creates the conditions in which ritual can occur naturally, respecting cultural, spiritual, and individual preferences.

Memory and personal items reinforce ecosystem dynamics. Shelves, tables, and alcoves provide space for photographs, religious symbols, or cherished objects. Their placement encourages interaction without crowding the room, offering tangible anchors for emotional connection. Objects interact with human behavior, creating opportunities for storytelling, reflection, and shared presence.

Flow through the room is influenced by multiple, simultaneous actors: patients, family members, staff, and volunteers. Micro-zones, unobstructed pathways, and subtle visual cues allow these actors to coexist harmoniously. The room manages human density without explicit signage, using proportion, furniture, and lighting to communicate rules of engagement intuitively.

The ecosystem concept also encompasses emotional regulation. Patients and family members experience stress, anxiety, and fatigue; the room's materials, lighting, and spatial organization function as stabilizers, mitigating emotional volatility. Even the smallest interventions—soft flooring, accessible seating, and gentle textures—affect perception and behavior, subtly guiding attention, posture, and engagement.

Spatial hierarchy supports behavioral ecology. Zones within the room—vigil, reflection, memory, and staff—interact dynamically, allowing human activity to occur without interference. The hierarchy communicates implicit boundaries, permitting intimacy while providing unobtrusive support for staff interventions. It also fosters autonomy for patients and visitors, reinforcing dignity and control.

Ultimately, the hospice room as ecosystem embodies the principle that architecture is active, not passive. It coexists with, anticipates, and shapes human behavior. Care is not solely a function of people; it is a choreography between space, materials, light, objects, and human presence. By designing with ecological intelligence, the quiet room sustains dignity, supports ritual, and provides a tangible structure for the intangible processes of grief, connection, and end-of-life transition.

This chapter previewed themes explored in later chapters: how objects, light, and ritual function within micro-zones; how tactile materials and textures influence engagement; and how architecture integrates with human activity to create an emotionally responsive, supportive environment. Understanding the room as ecosystem lays the foundation for examining these elements in greater depth.

2

The Emotional Architecture of Light

Light is far more than a functional necessity in hospice care; it is a medium that shapes emotional, physiological, and cognitive experience. The quality, intensity, direction, and color of illumination influence how patients perceive their environment, how family members interact, and even how staff deliver care. Scientific research confirms that light directly affects cortisol levels, circadian rhythms, and emotional states, meaning that architectural decisions regarding illumination carry tangible consequences for patient well-being.[1] In hospice care, where emotional fragility is heightened and physical vulnerability is acute, light is an essential instrument of comfort and psychological support.

Cortisol, the primary hormone regulating stress, is highly sensitive to light exposure. Bright, cool light during daytime hours promotes alertness and stabilizes circadian patterns, whereas warmer, dimmer light in the evening reduces arousal and fosters relaxation. Patients nearing the end of life often experience disrupted sleep–wake cycles and heightened sensitivity to environmental stimuli; properly designed lighting can support temporal orientation, reduce nighttime anxiety, and mitigate agitation that might otherwise occur during the vulnerable hours of evening or night. Light becomes both a physiological regulator and an emotional anchor, subtly guiding the body's internal clock while providing reassurance.

Overhead fluorescent lighting, historically ubiquitous in hospitals, is particularly ill-suited to hospice environments. Fluorescent tubes often produce glare, sharp shadows, and a sense of impersonality, all of which can exacerbate anxiety or trigger sensory discomfort. These harsh overhead sources create associations with sterility, illness, and institutional authority, evoking emotional responses that are antithetical to the goals of palliative care. For patients and families entering a hospice room, the first impression of cold, clinical illumination can undermine the delicate atmosphere of safety, dignity, and calm that the space is meant to convey.

Patients with cognitive vulnerabilities, including dementia or terminal agitation, are acutely affected by lighting quality. Sudden shifts in brightness or the presence of strong shadows can provoke fear, disorientation, or behavioral disturbances commonly known as sundowning. Shadows may be misinterpreted as threatening objects, creating distress that disrupts both patient and family presence. In contrast, consistent, evenly distributed illumination supports orientation, emotional regulation, and confidence in movement, helping patients inhabit the room safely without visual confusion.[2]

Adjustable, tunable lighting is a critical strategy for aligning illumination with the emotional climate of the room. Dimmers, variable color temperatures, and zoned lighting systems allow caregivers to tailor the environment to specific activities, moods, or times of day. For instance, a bedside lamp can be subtly brightened to facilitate a family vigil or gradually dimmed to create a tranquil setting for reflection and rest. Tunable lighting respects the fluidity of hospice care, allowing the environment to respond dynamically to human presence and emotional intensity.

The benefits of thoughtfully designed lighting extend beyond the patient to encompass family members and staff. Families often report feeling more at ease and emotionally attuned to the patient in softly illuminated environments, while staff benefit from lighting that allows precise care without creating visual intrusion or discomfort. By mediating visibility, mood, and relational tone, light functions as an unseen facilitator of interaction, guiding behavior and shaping experience without explicit intervention.

Natural light offers profound psychological and physiological benefits. Sunlight provides dynamic variation in intensity and color, reinforcing circadian cues and temporal orientation. Views framed by windows connect patients to the outside world, providing visual relief and reinforcing continuity with daily life. Architectural strategies such as light shelves, translucent curtains, or angled window openings modulate direct sunlight, preventing glare while preserving the benefits of natural illumination. This subtle interplay between daylight and interior space enhances both mental and emotional well-being.

Artificial light, when carefully selected, can replicate the beneficial qualities of natural light while supporting functional needs. Warm light-emitting diode (LED) sources with high color-rendering indices reduce harshness and preserve visual fidelity, making faces, objects, and surroundings appear more natural. Diffused light prevents high-contrast shadows that may disorient patients, fostering a consistent and calming visual environment. By harmonizing light with materiality, hospice rooms achieve a balance between visual comfort, aesthetic warmth, and functional clarity.

The direction of light is as important as its intensity. Low-level, indirect lighting minimizes shadows on the patient's face and body, reducing perceptual stress while creating a sense of intimacy. Downward-focused overhead lights, by contrast, can produce deep shadows and an unsettling visual atmosphere, accentuating features or contours that may provoke anxiety. Strategic positioning of side lighting, backlit panels, or concealed LED strips ensures that illumination supports both functional and emotional objectives.

Effective lighting balances procedural visibility with emotional sensitivity. Staff must perform essential tasks—medication administration, vital checks, and wound care—while minimizing intrusion into the patient's experience. Task lighting that is localized, adjustable, and non-glaring allows these procedures to occur without disrupting the overall atmosphere. The room's illumination thus fulfills dual functions: supporting clinical work while maintaining a calm, dignified environment for patients and families alike.

Color temperature is a powerful emotional cue. Cool, blue-toned light energizes and promotes alertness during daytime hours, whereas warm, amber light signals relaxation and facilitates calm in the evening. Tunable lighting systems enable gradual transitions that mirror natural circadian rhythms, providing temporal orientation and supporting the body's internal clock. This attention to color temperature reinforces both emotional regulation and physiological stability.

Shadows, reflections, and high-contrast surfaces must be carefully managed to prevent disorientation. Uneven lighting or reflective materials can create perceived obstacles or threatening shapes, particularly for patients with cognitive impairment or visual sensitivity. Matte surfaces, diffused illumination, and subtle color variation mitigate these effects, producing an environment that is visually coherent and psychologically stabilizing.

Nighttime lighting strategies are essential for safety and comfort. Patients often experience increased agitation, pain sensitivity, or confusion after dark. Low-level ambient illumination, soft nightlights, or bedside lamps provide sufficient visibility for safe movement and caregiving while minimizing disruption of sleep cycles. Gradual, nonintrusive lighting fosters a sense of security, reducing anxiety and supporting restful presence during vulnerable hours.

Light interacts synergistically with materials and surfaces. Warm wood, textured textiles, and matte walls diffuse illumination, softening harsh shadows and reflecting light gently across the room. Conversely, glossy or metallic surfaces amplify glare, heightening visual and emotional stress. Thoughtful alignment of materials and lighting enhances the room's capacity to convey care, calm, and psychological safety.

Task lighting for family engagement supports ritual, observation, and presence. Adjustable lamps allow reading, journaling, or intimate conversation without harsh illumination. Families can participate in caregiving or reflective practice while maintaining a sensory environment conducive to emotional regulation and prolonged presence. This empowers loved ones to remain fully engaged without fatigue or distraction.

The cumulative effect of carefully calibrated lighting on neuropsychology is substantial. Cortisol regulation, visual comfort, emotional stability, and circadian entrainment converge to influence mood, stress levels, and cognitive clarity.

Light becomes an active instrument in shaping the patient's perception of safety, dignity, and temporal orientation, extending beyond function to emotional care.

Lighting also serves as a form of symbolic communication. Gentle illumination signals attention, presence, and intentionality, while shadows, depth, and direction subtly define zones of interaction. Nonverbal cues embedded in the environment reinforce trust and support relational dynamics, providing reassurance when words may be inadequate.

Advances in lighting technology allow for increasingly nuanced control. Automated circadian systems, programmable dimmers, and zoned illumination provide staff with the ability to anticipate patient needs and adjust environmental conditions seamlessly. These technological interventions exemplify how architecture and infrastructure can actively support care, responding dynamically to human presence and emotional nuance.

Light anchors human ritual in the hospice room. Vigils, prayers, reading, reflection, and quiet conversation are all enhanced by thoughtful illumination. Gradual transitions in brightness, color, and direction allow rituals to unfold naturally, reinforcing the room's role as both a functional space and a container for meaning.

By understanding light as a neuropsychological and emotional instrument rather than a neutral utility, hospice designers create environments that respect circadian biology, emotional vulnerability, and relational dynamics. Light is not merely decoration or functionality; it is a form of care—an active participant in the choreography of presence, attention, and compassionate human connection.

Layered illumination is the cornerstone of a hospice room's emotional architecture. Light, when organized into multiple tiers, shapes not only visibility but also perception, mood, and relational dynamics. The three-tier strategy—ambient, task, and accent—allows designers to create an environment that simultaneously supports functional needs, emotional comfort, and spiritual resonance. Each layer interacts with the others, producing subtle gradations of brightness that guide attention, comfort the senses, and structure the emotional rhythms of presence.

Ambient lighting forms the foundation of layered illumination. This general, diffused light fills the room without drawing attention to itself, establishing a consistent baseline of visibility. In hospice design, ambient light is carefully calibrated to avoid glare, harsh shadows, or overly bright surfaces. Soft, indirect sources—concealed LEDs, diffused panels, or reflected light off walls and ceilings—create an environment that feels naturally luminous and psychologically supportive. Ambient light anchors spatial orientation, reducing visual stress and allowing patients and families to navigate the room intuitively.

Task lighting operates in tandem with ambient illumination, providing focused visibility for specific activities. Bedside lamps, reading lights, or movable floor lamps allow family members and caregivers to perform actions—such as administering medications, reading aloud, or holding vigil—without overwhelming the patient's visual field. The design of task lighting considers both intensity and direction, avoiding harsh shadows on the face and ensuring that illumination supports relational intimacy as well as functional clarity.

Accent lighting adds a third layer, transforming surfaces, objects, and zones into areas of focus or calm. Small lamps, concealed wall lights, or undershelf illumination create "glow pockets"—localized areas of gentle light that encourage reflection, ritual, or quiet interaction. Glow pockets are especially valuable for creating private corners within the hospice room, allowing visitors to engage in contemplative practice or personal connection without feeling exposed or intrusive. These illuminated micro-zones are psychologically reassuring, offering a sense of agency and sanctuary within the broader environment.

Bedside illumination requires particular attention, especially in the context of family presence and farewell. Light that gently warms facial expressions enhances the perception of closeness, comfort, and human connection. Shadows that obscure the patient's features or produce stark contrasts are avoided, as they can undermine emotional presence during moments of intense relational significance. Careful design ensures that family members can see and engage with the patient fully while preserving the room's overall calm and gentle aesthetic.

Partially illuminated rooms at night can cultivate a sense of sacred quiet. By leaving ambient light at low levels and selectively activating task or accent layers, the room achieves a balance between visibility and darkness. This subtle interplay communicates emotional permission for rest, reflection, and intimate presence. The human mind interprets these gentle gradations of light as nonintrusive, reinforcing feelings of safety, control, and reverence during the most vulnerable hours.

Light placement and shielding are crucial to prevent disturbing delicate sleep. Adjustable fixtures, diffusers, and indirect light sources ensure that illumination supports visibility without interrupting rest. Small, strategically positioned lights allow caregivers to attend to patient needs during night hours while minimizing circadian disruption or sensory intrusion. Such design choices reduce anxiety, facilitate uninterrupted rest, and maintain a sense of sacred containment within the room.

The choreography of layered light also interacts with spatial zones. Vigil areas, reflection corners, and memory shelves are illuminated selectively, guiding attention without imposing hierarchy or rigid control. Subtle differentiation of brightness communicates functional cues while preserving an overall emotional coherence, allowing human behavior to flow naturally within the room.

Color temperature plays a complementary role. Warm light reinforces intimacy and relaxation, while neutral or slightly cool task lighting ensures sufficient clarity for action. Accent lighting can introduce subtle shifts in hue to create visual interest, emphasize meaningful objects, or support ritualistic engagement. By integrating these variations, layered illumination becomes a dynamic participant in shaping perception, mood, and emotional tone.

Dimmer controls and programmable lighting systems further enhance flexibility. Caregivers can adjust the environment to match patient needs, visitation schedules, or circadian timing. These systems allow nuanced transitions between waking, reflective, and vigil periods, maintaining consistency and reducing abrupt visual shifts that might unsettle patients or visitors.

Indirect light, reflected off walls or ceilings, softens the environment and reduces visual stress. By bouncing light rather than directing it straight at occupants, designers create an ambient glow that is perceptually easier to inhabit. This technique minimizes glare, enhances spatial depth, and fosters a calming atmosphere that aligns with hospice goals of comfort and dignity.

Accent and glow pockets also serve as anchors for memory and ritual. Illuminated shelves for photographs, mementos, or religious symbols draw attention subtly without overwhelming the space. Light highlights the objects' presence, supporting emotional engagement, reflection, and family storytelling while maintaining the room's overall serenity.

Shadows are managed with deliberate care. Rather than erasing them completely, designers use soft gradations to communicate depth and structure while avoiding stark contrasts that might provoke anxiety. Shadows cast gently across textured surfaces or textiles contribute to a sense of dimension, making the room feel alive without disturbing its peaceful character.

Layered lighting contributes to relational dynamics. Family members feel permitted to sit close, read, or engage in rituals without the need to adjust overhead fixtures or strain their eyes. Staff can perform clinical interventions discreetly, blending care with emotional presence. In this way, illumination mediates human behavior, supporting both functional and psychological needs simultaneously.

Lighting zones are deliberately aligned with spatial micro-zones. Reflection corners receive soft accent light, memory shelves glow gently, and bedside areas benefit from adjustable task illumination. This orchestration ensures that the room accommodates multiple, overlapping human activities without visual conflict or cognitive overload.

Even minimal interventions, such as a single lamp or a shaded nightlight, significantly influence perception. Subtle cues communicated through light placement and intensity reduce stress, signal safety, and provide reassurance.

The cumulative impact of small, thoughtful interventions demonstrates the power of layered illumination in creating an emotionally responsive environment.

Technological integration enhances flexibility and adaptability. Programmable systems allow for automated transitions aligned with circadian rhythms, visitation schedules, or procedural needs. Light becomes an active agent, responding to human presence, time of day, and emotional intensity, rather than remaining a static environmental feature.

Ultimately, layered illumination transforms the hospice room from a purely functional space into a multidimensional, emotionally resonant environment. It supports human behavior, facilitates ritual, and communicates care through subtle gradations of brightness, hue, and direction. Light becomes both functional and symbolic, guiding attention, supporting relationships, and creating a sense of sacred containment for patients, families, and caregivers alike.

By sculpting atmosphere with ambient, task, and accent layers, hospice designers can create a room that supports emotional presence, relational intimacy, and physiological comfort simultaneously. Layered illumination is an invisible caregiver, responding to human need, mediating perception, and fostering an environment in which both life and memory are honored.[3]

Natural light is one of the most powerful instruments in hospice architecture, carrying both physiological and emotional weight. The placement of windows, the quality of light that enters the room, and its interaction with artificial sources determine how patients perceive time, space, and their own presence within the day's cycle. Proper integration of natural and artificial illumination establishes a visual and temporal rhythm that supports circadian health, emotional orientation, and relational engagement.

Window placement is a critical consideration. Patients should be able to orient themselves to the passage of the day, yet without experiencing glare or direct intrusion into sensitive visual fields. Strategically placed windows, often at eye level for patients who remain in bed, provide access to natural cues about sunrise, noon, and sunset, enhancing temporal awareness and reducing disorientation. The room thus becomes a medium through which the patient is subtly connected to the wider world, even as physical mobility declines.

Sunlight, when unfiltered, can be harsh and disorienting. Direct beams striking the eyes or the patient's face may provoke discomfort, headaches, or stress. Designers mitigate this through translucent curtains, light-diffusing glass, or adjustable louvers, ensuring that daylight is gentle, even, and psychologically soothing. In hospice care, in which the patient's sensitivity is heightened, careful modulation of natural light is as important as its availability.

Skylights and clerestory windows expand the possibilities of controlled natural light. These elevated sources provide daylight without the risk of direct glare, introducing a soft, diffuse quality that reaches the room uniformly. The shifting angle of sunlight throughout the day creates subtle patterns of illumination, enriching the environment with visual texture and providing cues for temporal orientation. Filtered skylights can also enhance mood, supporting reflection, connection, and the sense of spatial expansiveness.

Artificial light complements natural illumination, bridging periods of darkness or overcast weather. Tuned to match the spectral quality and warmth of daylight, artificial sources maintain continuity in visual perception and emotional tone. This integration ensures that patients experience consistent lighting cues throughout the day, preserving circadian rhythms and supporting emotional stability, even when natural light is absent.

Timed lighting transitions enhance the perceptual rhythm of the day. Gradually dimming lights in the evening or shifting color temperature to warmer tones signals approaching rest or reflection. Families benefit from these transitions as well, intuitively understanding the rhythm of daily life and participating in rituals, prayers, or reflection in synchrony with natural cycles. This subtle choreography of light frames emotional presence and relational timing without verbal direction.

The emotional effect of witnessing sunrise or sunset from a hospice bed is profound. These daily phenomena connect patients to the continuity of the world outside their immediate experience, reinforcing a sense of life's natural cadence. Families often describe moments of watching dawn or dusk together as deeply meaningful, creating shared memories that transcend the clinical setting and highlight the sacredness of everyday time.

Light directionality must be carefully considered to enhance comfort. Windows facing strong morning or afternoon sun are often fitted with vertical blinds, sheer curtains, or adjustable shades to diffuse intensity while preserving brightness. The goal is to prevent direct intrusion into the patient's line of sight while maintaining connection with the outside world, supporting both physiological and emotional well-being.

Integration of natural and artificial light must also account for shadows and visual contrasts. Harsh sunlight can cast deep shadows that exaggerate objects or create visual confusion. By layering artificial sources—ambient, task, and accent—designers smooth these contrasts, providing stable illumination while preserving the dynamism and richness that daylight brings.

The interplay of light and materials enhances this relationship. Reflective surfaces, warm woods, and textured textiles diffuse both natural and artificial light, softening its impact and amplifying its emotional effect. Walls and ceilings can act as secondary light sources, reflecting sunlight into shadowed areas and maintaining a balanced visual field. This thoughtful orchestration transforms the room into a living canvas, responsive to both environmental and human factors.

Orientation to seasonal changes is another benefit of daylight integration. Exposure to shifting sunlight angles, color temperatures, and brightness throughout the year provides natural markers of temporal progression. Patients experience subtle cues of seasons passing, reinforcing continuity with the external environment and mitigating the sense of isolation that can accompany long-term hospice care.

Artificial light systems can be programmed to mimic these seasonal variations, complementing natural cues and maintaining perceptual continuity. Gradual shifts in intensity or hue simulate dawn, noon, and dusk, reinforcing circadian alignment and emotional stability. These nuanced lighting strategies extend the benefits of natural light even in enclosed or urban settings in which window access is limited.

Layered illumination allows natural and artificial sources to coexist harmoniously. Ambient daylight forms the base layer; task lighting provides clarity where needed; and accent illumination highlights zones for reflection, ritual, or memory. Together, these layers respond dynamically to human presence and activity, adapting to visitation schedules, caregiving tasks, or moments of intimacy without compromising comfort.

The emotional resonance of light is amplified through deliberate visual framing. Views of trees, sky, or gardens through windows connect patients to natural cycles and evoke a sense of peace. Even partially obstructed or filtered views maintain psychological continuity, reinforcing the patient's awareness of time, weather, and the broader environment beyond the room.

In the evening, low-level artificial light maintains orientation while preserving a sense of calm. By carefully calibrating brightness and color temperature, designers create a protective cocoon that allows patients to rest, families to remain present, and caregivers to perform tasks unobtrusively. The room thus supports multiple human needs simultaneously without compromising emotional tone.

Careful balance between natural and artificial light also supports nocturnal vigilance. Subtle illumination near the bedside or along pathways ensures that staff can attend to patients safely, while low-level ambient light prevents startling contrasts that might disrupt sleep or provoke anxiety. This integration honors both functional and emotional priorities, creating a room that is responsive, adaptable, and reassuring.

Light-mediated rituals are central to hospice experience. Morning reflection in soft daylight, afternoon reading under diffuse illumination, and evening vigil in warm artificial light provide temporal anchors that structure presence and emotional engagement. Layered integration allows these rituals to unfold naturally, supporting both patient autonomy and family participation.

The room's design anticipates variability in light conditions. Cloud cover, seasonal shifts, and architectural obstructions affect natural light availability; artificial sources are carefully calibrated to fill gaps without overwhelming or confusing the patient. This adaptability ensures that the emotional and functional qualities of light remain consistent, maintaining continuity of care and presence.

Ultimately, the dance between natural and artificial light is an intricate choreography that balances physiological need, emotional comfort, and relational intimacy. When executed thoughtfully, the interplay fosters a sense of temporal orientation, continuity with the outside world, and psychological safety. The hospice room becomes a responsive environment, capable of supporting the complexity of human presence at life's end.

By integrating daylight with tunable artificial systems, designers craft a room in which the passage of time, emotional rhythms, and human connection are made visible and tangible. Light is no longer merely functional; it is an active participant in the hospice experience, shaping memory, supporting rituals, and nurturing dignity in the most fragile moments.

Dimming light in a hospice room is far more than an aesthetic or functional act; it is a form of communication, a subtle cue that signals the sacredness of time and presence. In many hospices, the act of lowering light levels before intimate conversations or family gatherings is experienced as an unspoken permission to engage emotionally, to attend fully to the patient, and to prepare for moments of transition. This practice transforms the room into a stage for human connection, with light functioning as both medium and message.

The nurse's hand on a dimmer switch is often the first gesture that announces intentionality. Gradually lowering the ambient light signals the onset of a vigil, an intimate period in which the patient, family, and caregivers are invited to pause, reflect, or speak from the heart. This transition is subtle yet psychologically potent, establishing a temporal container for attention and presence. The dimming process itself becomes a ritual, an embodied reminder that what follows is sacred and carefully observed.

Bedside lamps play a central role in these rituals. A softly glowing lamp near the patient's head provides a focused pool of light that illuminates faces without flooding the room with brightness. Families intuitively gather near this "light island," and the small circle of illumination fosters closeness, conversation, and the subtle transmission of care. The lamp's glow is comforting, creating a safe visual environment while emphasizing the patient as the center of attention.

The ritual of dimming light also structures the rhythm of the day. Evening hours are often associated with reflection, prayer, or vigil, and the transition from higher ambient light to softer illumination prepares the psyche for quiet presence. These transitions are carefully timed and executed gradually to avoid abrupt sensory disruption, allowing the patient and family to experience continuity and psychological ease.

In the final hours of life, dimming light carries symbolic weight. The gradual lowering of illumination communicates respect, reverence, and attention, framing the patient's last moments with dignity. Families often describe a profound emotional resonance during these periods, noting that the quality of light shapes memory and creates a sense of closure even before verbal farewells are spoken.

The bedside lamp ritual extends to the moments after death. Turning off the lamp once the patient has passed functions as a symbolic act of closure. It communicates that the immediate presence of care has concluded, while leaving the room in a gentle, restorative darkness that supports mourning, reflection, and the initial stages of grieving. This ritual acknowledges the emotional significance of light as a medium of attention and care.

Warm, flickering light, whether from LEDs or filtered incandescent sources, often evokes the cultural metaphor of candlelight. Safe alternatives to open flame—such as battery-powered or warm LED candles—allow ritualistic lighting without compromising safety. These small sources of light serve as visual markers of attention, presence, and reverence, creating micro-rituals that reinforce the sacred character of hospice care.

Cultural and religious traditions provide frameworks for understanding light as a spiritual signal. In Jewish practice, the shabbat candles, yahrzeit candles, or other ceremonial lightings create temporal markers of reflection, memory, and sacred presence. In Buddhist traditions, soft light and ritualized illumination mark periods of meditation, mindfulness, or preparation for transition. Catholic and Christian practices incorporate candles or dimmed light to emphasize prayer, reflection, and the sacredness of life's passage. Indigenous practices often use light symbolically to honor ancestors, natural cycles, or the passage between life and death. These cultural frameworks inform hospice design, allowing light rituals to resonate meaningfully with diverse patients and families.

The emotional impact of dimming rituals is amplified by anticipation. As ambient light gradually lowers, the mind senses a transition in time and attention. Heart rate, breathing, and cognitive arousal often subtly adjust in response, producing a physiological cue that aligns with the emotional intent of the ritual. Light becomes a bridge between external environment and internal emotional state, guiding presence without words.

Families often internalize these cues, entering the space with a heightened sense of reverence or preparedness. The rhythm of dimming frames behavior and focus, allowing loved ones to approach the patient with tenderness and intentionality. In this way, architectural and technological elements become agents of relational support, shaping behavior, emotion, and memory simultaneously.

The spatial distribution of light reinforces these effects. Glow pockets around memory shelves, bedside lamps, or seating areas create zones of intimacy that correspond with ritual behavior. These micro-zones allow multiple rituals—quiet conversation, prayer, and reflection—to occur concurrently without visual or emotional interference. The careful orchestration of these illuminated areas supports diverse needs while maintaining overall room harmony.

The interplay of dimmed light with shadow is also psychologically significant. Shadows cast softly across walls or textiles introduce visual depth without harsh contrast, reinforcing the sense of calm and continuity. This interplay enhances perceptual comfort while subtly emphasizing spatial boundaries and relational zones. Shadows, rather than being eliminated, are harnessed as tools for emotional and spatial orientation.

Staff involvement in light-based rituals fosters shared meaning. Caregivers who dim lights or adjust glow pockets actively participate in the emotional choreography of the room, aligning their presence with patient and family rhythms. This integration of human action and environmental design strengthens the relational fabric of hospice care, creating a collaborative experience of attention and presence.

Light rituals also provide memory cues for families. Photographs, mementos, or personal objects illuminated during dimmed periods are experienced with heightened emotional salience. These associations persist beyond the immediate moment, contributing to enduring recollections of care, intimacy, and shared attention during the patient's final days.

Even small gestures, such as activating a bedside lamp or adjusting a shade, carry symbolic resonance. In the context of hospice, every manipulation of light communicates intention, attention, and respect. The act of controlling illumination becomes a silent language of care, comprehensible to those present even in the absence of verbal explanation.

Lighting can also accommodate cultural or personal adaptation. Patients or families may request certain colors, brightness levels, or ritual patterns aligned with personal beliefs. Hospices that incorporate flexible lighting systems allow these preferences to be realized, reinforcing the patient's dignity and the family's engagement in meaningful ritual.

Technological sophistication enhances the potential for these practices. Dimmer switches, programmable LEDs, and localized glow pockets allow staff to create nuanced sequences of illumination. Automated circadian-based systems can gradually lower light in alignment with day–night cycles, supporting both physiological and emotional transitions without requiring constant manual adjustment.

These rituals are not merely symbolic; they have measurable psychological effects. Research indicates that subtle, intentional changes in ambient light influence arousal, stress, and perceived safety. In the hospice context, dimming can reduce agitation, support calm reflection, and enhance relational presence, demonstrating the tangible benefits of integrating ritualized light practices into environmental design.

Finally, light-based rituals cultivate a sense of sacred time within the hospice room. By signaling transitions, framing presence, and highlighting relational focus, dimming elevates ordinary environmental manipulation into a form of caregiving. Patients, families, and staff experience light as both medium and message, creating enduring emotional resonance that shapes memory, honors life, and supports the profound intimacy of the final days.

Through the deliberate orchestration of dimming and glow, the hospice environment becomes a participant in care. Light communicates, structures, and sanctifies the passage of time, reinforcing human presence and emotional connection. It is a ritualized act, a bridge between life and memory, offering both practical guidance and symbolic meaning in the delicate, sacred moments of hospice care.

The moments following death are emotionally charged, steeped in grief, presence, and ritual, and in these fragile intervals the role of lighting becomes far more than functional. In hospice rooms, illumination acts as an integral participant in the emotional choreography, guiding attention gently, supporting dignity with intention, and shaping the atmosphere in a way that allows families to feel both seen and held. Softened, carefully layered lighting communicates a depth of care that words cannot, signaling respect for both the deceased and the grieving, and offering a visual environment that sustains emotional focus without intruding on the intimacy of the moment.

Family arrival after a patient's passing often marks the first encounter with a space that feels both familiar and irrevocably changed. Soft ambient light immediately conveys calm, containment, and a subtle invitation to breathe. Harsh overhead lighting can cast the room in a clinical or abrupt tone, creating a sense of intrusion, whereas subdued, evenly distributed illumination establishes a quiet reverence that helps families orient themselves. When loved ones enter a dimmed, warm environment, they intuitively perceive it as a space designed to honor grief, memory, and the delicate transition taking place.

Task lighting during postmortem care is another essential element that must be handled with nuance. Staff performing body preparation or cleansing require sufficient visibility to ensure hygiene and safety, yet illumination must remain subtle enough to preserve the dignity of the deceased and the emotional well-being of the family. Diffused, directional lighting—such as movable lamps with warm filters—creates a balance in which clinical needs are met without generating a harsh, dehumanizing field of brightness. In this way, light becomes a tool of care, reflecting a deliberate blending of practical necessity with emotional sensitivity.

Illumination also serves as a mediator of emotional tone, modulating the room's affective landscape through shifts in intensity or warmth. These subtle adjustments guide family members' experience, signaling that the central focus is presence rather than procedural activity. Small pools of gentle glow around personal mementos, bedside photographs, or floral arrangements create visual anchors that reinforce relational memory, offering points of meaning within the room while avoiding the stark, impersonal feel that overhead light can impose.

Cultural and religious differences further necessitate flexible, adaptable lighting strategies. Some traditions call for brighter illumination to signify celebration, ritual cleansing, or active participation in the transition, whereas others prefer muted, contemplative light that aligns with practices of quiet reflection. Hospices that incorporate adjustable, tunable lighting systems can respond to these varied preferences, ensuring that the environment supports meaningful ritual without compromise and allows every family to experience care that resonates with their beliefs.

Objects within the hospice room are transformed by intentional illumination into emotional anchors that deepen connection. A softly lit photograph, a cherished book, or a religious symbol becomes a focal point for memory and reflection, with the interplay of shadow and glow enhancing texture, depth, and presence. This visual treatment subtly reinforces the continuity of care and the narrative of the patient's life. These objects—bathed in gentle, purposeful light—preserve relational memory long after the immediate moment has faded, creating a sense of continuity for families navigating early grief.

The choreography of light during family gatherings also shapes the flow of behavior in the room. Areas intended for sitting, reflection, and conversation are illuminated softly, guiding attention toward zones of presence while maintaining overall cohesion. Task or accent lights subtly mark ritual areas, offering guidance without imposing hierarchy or drawing focus away from shared moments. Through this gentle hierarchy, simultaneous activities such as quiet conversation, silent reflection, and ritual practice can unfold harmoniously in the same space.

Warmth in lighting temperature plays a crucial role in supporting emotional regulation. Amber and soft yellow hues foster calmness, reduce physiological arousal, and create a sense of relational intimacy that is difficult to achieve in cooler tones. Families consistently report that warm lighting feels emotionally safe and nurturing, helping mitigate the harshness often associated with medical environments. In contrast, cooler or neutral lighting may introduce a sense of detachment or sterility, diminishing the room's ability to hold grief gently.

Glow pockets and accent illumination also guide temporal perception, offering visual cues that help families understand when reflection, prayer, or private conversation may be appropriate. Light communicates subtle changes in attention and presence, functioning as an unspoken guide through moments that can feel overwhelming. These cues help coordinate behaviors without verbal instruction, supporting families in making intuitive choices during emotionally charged experiences.

The act of dimming lights as a farewell ritual serves as a visual metaphor for closure, connecting the sensory environment to the emotional transition at hand. Gradually lowering ambient and task illumination creates a space in which the act of goodbye can unfold with a sense of reverence and intentionality. This soft transition resonates across cultures and emotional states, giving form to the unspoken acknowledgment that presence is shifting, and offering families a symbolic gesture of completion and respect.

Shadows are managed with equal intentionality to preserve depth without creating discomfort. Soft, directional light allows family members to perceive the room clearly while preventing the deep contrasts that may amplify emotional distress. The interplay of light and shadow provides spatial orientation, emotional containment, and visual interest simultaneously, ensuring that the environment remains soothing without becoming visually flattened or stark.

Artificial lighting must also respond seamlessly to variations in natural light. Overcast days, limited windows, or evening hours require subtle supplementation to maintain warmth and consistency. Tunable LEDs, concealed strips, and movable lamps allow staff to preserve the emotional tone of the room regardless of external conditions, ensuring that light consistently supports presence rather than disrupting it.

Light also guides the movements and behavior of staff during grief-sensitive moments. Caregivers adjust intensity to signal their availability, support procedures with dignity, and respect the rhythms of family rituals. These small gestures, although easily overlooked, shape the relational atmosphere of the room and ensure that the environment aligns with both human and procedural needs.

The interplay of ambient, task, and accent lighting establishes a gentle hierarchy of visual attention. Families naturally gravitate toward the patient, personal mementos, and designated ritual areas, while peripheral zones remain softly illuminated to maintain spatial coherence. This subtle hierarchy reinforces emotional prioritization without requiring verbal cues, revealing the nuanced role that lighting plays in shaping perception and experience.

Memory formation is deeply influenced by illumination, especially during moments of emotional significance. Research suggests that events associated with subtle, warm lighting are encoded more vividly, which underscores the importance of visual context in shaping lasting recollection. Hospice designers leverage this phenomenon to enhance the memorial quality of the environment, helping families carry forward memories that feel grounded, coherent, and gently framed.

Candlelight metaphors—often realized through safe LEDs or diffused incandescent sources—continue to play a powerful role in ritual and reflection. These forms of illumination evoke cultural and spiritual associations with presence, attention, and sacredness, while avoiding safety risks. Families frequently gather near these lights, engaging in prayer, storytelling, or silent connection, with the glow shaping both physical proximity and emotional closeness.

Lighting adjustments often synchronize with auditory and tactile cues, creating a multisensory environment that supports presence and emotional regulation. Soft music, gentle footsteps, or the texture of warm textiles interact with light to form a landscape that reduces cognitive overload and preserves dignity. This holistic environment helps families navigate emotional intensity with greater grounding and ease.

Even the smallest lighting interventions—such as increasing a lamp's glow or easing it into dimness—communicate care and intentionality. Families often perceive these gestures as expressions of attentiveness, reinforcing trust and emotional safety. The hospice room becomes an active participant in human interaction, shaping atmosphere and meaning rather than serving as a neutral backdrop.

Ritualized use of light also supports post-death processing, helping families move through shock toward a sense of coherence. Families who witness intentional dimming, the creation of glow pockets, or careful lamp management often report a greater feeling of continuity, emotional regulation, and narrative closure. Light becomes a temporal marker for mourning, framing the earliest moments of grief as part of a larger arc of remembrance.

Finally, lighting design in these sacred moments exemplifies the integration of architecture, technology, and emotional insight. Hospices that thoughtfully calibrate illumination for grief, gathering, and goodbye create environments that honor life, uphold dignity, and support the complexity of human presence. In this context, light transcends mere function, becoming a medium of connection, memory, and care—one that continues to resonate long after the room returns to stillness.

3
Objects as Anchors of Presence

Objects in hospice rooms are never merely functional; they carry emotional weight, becoming silent participants in care, ritual, and the experience of presence itself. A water pitcher on a bedside table, a favorite blanket folded neatly at the foot of the bed, a familiar lamp casting a soft glow, or even a simple tissue box can acquire symbolic significance that far exceeds their practical purpose. These items anchor presence, evoke memory, and provide tactile and visual comfort for both patient and family, forming a constellation of meaning within the space. In a setting in which words are sometimes inadequate or exhausted, objects become a secondary language, communicating attention, gentleness, and dignity through their placement, condition, and the gestures they invite.

Consider the water pitcher. It is more than hydration; it represents attentiveness and readiness. When staff place a filled pitcher within easy reach, they silently communicate vigilance and care—an unspoken promise to meet needs promptly and respectfully. This simple object becomes a visual cue of presence and respect for autonomy, reminding families that the patient is being held in consistent regard. Families often interpret such items as tangible symbols that their loved one is not only seen but also valued, and even small rituals involving the pitcher—pouring a glass of water, adjusting a straw, or refilling it—carry profound symbolic weight that reinforces relational closeness and practical tenderness.

Blankets are another critical object, merging functionality with emotional resonance in ways that become increasingly powerful as the patient's condition changes. A folded quilt, a soft fleece, or a favorite throw embodies warmth, safety, and familiarity, serving as both a physical comfort and a symbolic gesture of protection. Families frequently use blankets to wrap the patient gently, symbolizing continuity, care, and tenderness even in moments when communication is limited. These textiles often evoke layers of memory—the scent of home, the tactile recall of past experiences, or the soothing rhythms of past routines—bringing comfort during moments of fear, agitation, or emotional intensity.

Tissues serve an unexpectedly emotional role within the hospice environment. Their presence anticipates vulnerability, grief, and tears, acknowledging the emotional reality of the space before words are spoken. Thoughtful placement of tissues communicates preparation and empathy, signaling that the hospice team and the room itself are ready to accommodate emotion without judgment or hesitation. When tissues are placed within arm's reach, the accessibility transforms this ordinary object into a small but potent ritual instrument, supporting both the immediate needs of grief and the broader emotional landscape of care.

Lighting objects, such as bedside lamps, function as anchors of relational attention and spatial coherence. A softly glowing lamp highlights zones for conversation, reflection, or prayer, subtly signaling where presence is focused and how interaction might unfold. Its placement communicates relational priority: The patient's presence remains central, even when attention shifts between individuals in the room. Family members often orient themselves by the glow, instinctively gathering near illuminated objects that gently guide human behavior, promote connection, and create boundaries of intimacy within the larger space.

The concept of "object-as-ritual" highlights how seemingly mundane actions acquire emotional and symbolic meaning in hospice settings. Brushing a patient's hair, smoothing a blanket, or pouring water from a pitcher becomes a visible manifestation of care, an embodied expression of love and attentiveness. These actions, although small in scale, carry significant emotional weight, transforming routine tasks into ritualized gestures that communicate continuity, dignity, and presence. In this way, objects become extensions of the caregiver's hand, enabling care that is both practical and profoundly symbolic.

Objects also provide continuity and support identity, especially in settings in which patients may feel that their sense of self is slipping away. A favorite mug on the bedside table may carry memories of daily rituals, preferred beverages, or comforting moments from earlier life chapters. In hospice, this mug becomes a symbol of persistence, personal choice, and narrative continuity—a reminder of who the patient is beyond illness or decline. Staff often position such items intentionally, ensuring they remain visible and accessible, reinforcing identity in ways that support emotional grounding and relational connection.

Staff awareness of object placement is deliberate, reflecting an understanding that every item contributes to the emotional architecture of the room. Objects are arranged not only for functional accessibility but also for their emotional impact, creating a spatial grammar of care through intentional alignment. A neatly positioned blanket, a tissue box placed thoughtfully within reach, or a personal photo displayed at eye level communicates care while reinforcing spatial coherence. This sensitivity transforms the room from a clinical site of care into a curated emotional environment that supports both ritual and presence.

Even small objects can serve as anchors for family interaction, shaping how loved ones gather, connect, and express care. A simple chair drawn close to the bedside, a soft pillow placed for comfort, or a small table designated for mementos enables families to establish proximity and enact relational rituals.

These objects scaffold human presence, mediating interactions and facilitating acts of love, attention, and memory. They create small zones in which gestures of connection unfold naturally and meaningfully.

Personal objects act as visual cues for stories and recollections, becoming catalysts for narrative continuity in moments when families seek grounding. A photograph, a small statue, or a handwritten note invites storytelling, prompting family members to recount moments of life, anecdotes, or shared memories that bring warmth into a difficult space. These items transform the room into a narrative environment in which memory is active, relational, and sustaining, bridging the patient's past with the intimacy of the present moment.

The tactile qualities of objects are equally significant, offering sensory grounding in moments when emotional experiences may feel overwhelming or disorienting. Smooth wood, soft fabric, cool metal, or textured ceramics communicate presence through touch, linking sensory engagement with emotional reassurance. Patients and family members often engage physically with these objects—holding, stroking, adjusting, or arranging them—as part of ritualized interaction. Tactile engagement reinforces the emotional significance of ordinary items, bridging sensory experience with memory, presence, and layers of relational meaning.

The emotional anthropology of hospice objects underscores how simple items can acquire sacred weight through use, intention, and ritual. Everyday objects, when incorporated into care or routine gestures, become symbols of attention, presence, and dignity. A folded blanket, a lined notepad, or a filled water pitcher is no longer mundane; it becomes embedded with meaning that reflects the emotional labor of caregiving and the relational depth of the hospice environment. These objects hold emotional charge precisely because they are touched repeatedly with intention.

Objects also help regulate the emotional rhythm of the room, guiding attention and modulating affective tones. Glow pockets, a dimmed lamp, or a softly scented candle work together to create zones of relational presence, delineating areas for reflection, conversation, or quiet attention. Families and caregivers orient themselves both spatially and emotionally around these cues, allowing moments of calm, reflection, or vigilance to unfold in the rhythm appropriate to the moment. Light interacts with objects to shape a quiet choreography of presence.

The integration of personal mementos ensures that the room reflects the patient's life rather than presenting as a neutral or exclusively institutional space. Jewelry, photographs, small sculptures, or cherished books provide both visual and tactile anchors that reinforce identity and continuity. These objects act as emotional bridges, linking the patient's lived experience to present care, reminding families and staff that the patient's story extends far beyond the bed and into a rich, meaningful life that continues to be honored.

Objects also serve as implicit instructions for behavior, offering gentle visual cues that guide how families and staff interact with the space. Chairs positioned close to the bedside, a lamp highlighting a memory shelf, or a pitcher placed within easy reach subtly communicate how to engage respectfully and attentively. Families intuitively follow these cues, performing rituals of care, presence, and connection without needing direct instruction. Through these objects, the room quietly teaches participants how to inhabit the space with reverence.

The patient's favorite mug, cup, or utensil often becomes emblematic of autonomy and persistence, especially during the final days of life. Staff ensure that such items are not only visible but also positioned in ways that reinforce identity and personal agency. Even when physical use becomes limited, these small objects maintain narrative continuity and support relational engagement by reminding everyone present of the patient's individuality, preferences, and enduring presence.

Lighting objects, such as adjustable bedside lamps, reinforce ritualized behavior by marking zones of intentional activity. Families naturally gather around softly illuminated areas for prayer, storytelling, reading, or silent companionship, and the placement, intensity, and warmth of light guide these moments with subtle clarity. In this way, objects function not only as anchors but also as beacons that signal sacred or meaningful interactions within the room's emotional landscape.

Objects also mediate the experience of grief, offering tangible points of engagement for family members navigating the complex emotional terrain of loss. Tissues, blankets, mementos, or ritual items provide a comforting interface between emotional intensity and the physical world, enabling family members to externalize feelings through touch, arrangement, or interaction. These gestures support psychological and relational needs, helping loved ones remain connected to the patient and each other as they process impending or recent loss.

Even minor interventions with objects communicate care and relational presence. Folding a blanket over a lap, placing a hand on a lamp switch to soften the glow, or arranging personal items with intention becomes a gesture of attentiveness that reinforces dignity. These small acts of adjustment scaffold human interaction, shaping moments of tenderness and signaling presence during each stage of hospice care.

Finally, the careful curation of objects transforms the hospice room into an emotionally coherent ecosystem in which meaning, memory, and presence converge. Objects, light, spatial arrangement, and materiality interact seamlessly to anchor presence, support ritual, and facilitate memory-making. Through thoughtful placement and use, the hospice room becomes a tangible manifestation of care, where attention, identity, and dignity are physically and symbolically reinforced, creating an environment that supports both the living and the dying with quiet depth.

Bedside tables, shelves, and small surfaces in hospice rooms serve as more than functional furniture; they become repositories of memory, ritual, and relational significance. Each item placed on these surfaces transforms the room into a narrative space, telling a story about the patient's life, personality, and relationships. A framed photograph, a small trinket, or a handwritten letter becomes a tangible representation of care, presence, and continuity, connecting the past, present, and impending absence in a highly emotionally resonant manner.[1]

These surfaces often function as temporary shrines, curated deliberately by family members, friends, and hospice staff. Each object placed on a table or shelf is imbued with symbolic significance: Photographs of children or grandchildren, cherished jewelry, favorite books, or personal mementos collectively communicate attention, respect, and acknowledgment of the patient's individuality. Through this curation, the hospice room becomes a sacred and emotionally layered environment, transforming ordinary space into a stage for reflection, interaction, and ritual.

Shelves provide the added advantage of verticality, creating layers of visual and emotional attention. By arranging objects at varying heights, designers and family members can establish zones of focus and intimacy. A small religious symbol at eye level invites contemplation and meditation, while a framed photograph or keepsake placed lower encourages tactile engagement and closer proximity. The vertical arrangement not only organizes the space visually but also structures relational and emotional attention within the room.

Family members often take an active role in curating these memory surfaces. Selecting, arranging, or rotating items becomes an act of love, care, and engagement. This curatorial process supports the family's grieving journey, allowing them to honor the patient's identity, celebrate milestones, and participate actively in the shaping of the hospice environment.[2] Each placement becomes a ritualized gesture, quietly reinforcing presence, attention, and relational continuity.

The concept of micro-altars is central to understanding these surfaces. A bedside table or shelf can serve as a concentrated zone of focus, where ritual, reflection, and emotional processing converge. The careful arrangement of objects—such as a small candle, a personal trinket, or a spiritual icon—creates a visual and symbolic focal point. Families naturally orient their presence around these micro-altars, allowing for silent reflection, prayer, or storytelling that honors both the patient and the relational network gathered around them.

Memory surfaces must balance personalization with functional clarity. Although it is important to allow meaningful objects to be displayed, surfaces must remain organized and uncluttered to reduce cognitive overload and maintain visual calm. Clear delineation of zones for different objects, combined with minimalist spatial design, ensures that personalization does not overwhelm the room, supporting psychological comfort for both patient and family.

Bedside tables often serve a dual purpose, blending functional and symbolic roles. A favorite mug, a water pitcher, or hand lotion may sit alongside photographs and mementos. These objects, although practical, gain additional meaning in their context, bridging daily care activities with symbolic gestures of attention, continuity, and love. This layering of function and meaning transforms ordinary tasks into emotionally resonant rituals.

Material choice is another important factor in the design of memory surfaces. Warm wood, textured laminates, or soft-finished metals invite tactile engagement, allowing family members to touch, hold, and interact with personal items meaningfully. These sensory qualities enhance emotional connection and support ritualized behavior, reinforcing principles of tactile and visual psychology in end-of-life care.[3]

Micro-altars and memory surfaces are particularly meaningful during vigil periods. Family members often gather near these surfaces to reflect, pray, or share memories. The objects act as visual and tactile cues, structuring attention and relational presence without verbal instruction. These surfaces guide human behavior and emotional focus, providing an accessible means of supporting intimacy, remembrance, and ritualized engagement.

After death, memory surfaces continue to hold significance. Objects left on tables and shelves act as transitional anchors, helping families navigate the immediate emotional aftermath. These items maintain continuity, offering a tangible link to the patient's identity and life story while allowing loved ones to process grief gradually before objects are returned home, moved, or otherwise rearranged.

Memory surfaces also serve as implicit guides for ritualized behavior. A carefully positioned photograph may prompt storytelling, while a small religious icon may guide prayer or reflection. These surfaces scaffold engagement, providing cues for how to interact meaningfully with the patient's memory and with one another, creating opportunities for relational intimacy even in the absence of the patient.

The spatial relationship between memory surfaces, bed, chairs, and light sources is intentional. Designers and staff use surface placement to create zones of focus, guiding families naturally toward areas of reflection and ritual. This intentional spatial choreography supports relational presence while maintaining functional accessibility and overall room coherence.

Arrangement of objects on these surfaces communicates narrative and identity. The careful sequencing of photos, letters, and personal items allows families to tell stories visually, layering meaning in ways that reinforce relational connection. A bedside table with photographs of grandchildren, a favorite book, and a trinket from travel communicate aspects of personality, history, and relationships, offering a sense of narrative continuity during the final days.

Staff play a key role in facilitating the arrangement and maintenance of memory surfaces. Nurses and aides often guide families in placing items safely, ensuring visibility, accessibility, and functional efficiency. This guidance helps preserve dignity and emotional resonance, integrating both practical and symbolic priorities within the hospice room.

The interplay of light and memory surfaces enhances their significance. Accent lighting, filtered natural light, or soft glow from a bedside lamp draws attention to curated objects without overwhelming the visual environment. Light transforms these surfaces into visual anchors, highlighting relational and emotional priorities in a subtle yet powerful manner.

Memory surfaces support multisensory engagement. Families can touch a smooth photo frame, stroke a textured blanket, or handle small ritual objects, combining tactile, visual, and olfactory input. These interactions strengthen memory, reinforce emotional connection, and provide a sense of intimacy, making the space emotionally rich and responsive to human needs.

The concept of transitional objects is also relevant after death. Memory surfaces, with objects left in place temporarily, provide continuity for families navigating grief. They allow for a measured separation from the patient, offering tangible points of focus to process loss while maintaining symbolic connection to identity, ritual, and shared memory.

Memory surfaces may also accommodate spiritual or cultural practices. Prayer beads, sacred texts, ritual candles, or symbolic figurines allow families to perform faith-based rituals without disrupting room functionality. Thoughtful placement of these items ensures accessibility, prominence, and emotional resonance, reinforcing the room's sacred character.

Ultimately, memory surfaces function as curated emotional landscapes, integrating personal artifacts, functional items, and ritual objects into coherent zones of attention, care, and reflection. They anchor presence, support relational engagement, and provide tangible means for families to enact care, perform ritual, and preserve memory, creating spaces that are both physically and emotionally meaningful.

Even in their modest scale, these surfaces carry extraordinary significance. They mediate human interaction, reinforce dignity, and provide continuity across the transition from life to memory. Thoughtful attention to memory surfaces is a cornerstone of hospice design, demonstrating how objects, placement, and relational intent converge to create profound emotional impact.

The chair by the window is more than a seat; it is a place of devotion, witness, and presence—a quiet sanctuary for those who remain attentive during the most vulnerable hours of life. Across cultures and histories, the act of sitting vigil has long been recognized as a sacred gesture—watching over the dying, guarding the passage from life to death, and providing an embodied space in which reflection, prayer, and attentive presence naturally emerge. In modern hospice design, the window chair fulfills both symbolic and practical roles, becoming a throne of vigilance where family, friends, and caregivers participate in the profound and humbling act of bearing witness. Its placement and design reinforce the gravity of the moment, supporting the kind of stillness and presence that words alone cannot provide.

The history of the vigil chair is long and varied, reflecting a cross-cultural understanding that the dying should not be left alone. In medieval Europe, bedside chairs were positioned intentionally for attendants who remained close to the patient to ensure warmth, companionship, and spiritual presence during final hours. In Japanese and other Eastern traditions, low, wide chairs or mats were placed near windows to encourage meditation, prayer, and quiet reflection as one prepared to transition from life to death. These historical precedents inform modern hospice design, reminding us that the need for a dedicated space to observe, reflect, and connect transcends time and geography. The modern window chair carries the weight of these traditions, preserving a lineage of care within contemporary practice.

Psychologically, the vigil chair provides a retreat spot within the hospice room, offering family members a sense of personal space while still allowing them to remain proximate to the patient. The chair functions as a buffer from the emotional intensity of the bedside, giving watchers a place to regulate their emotions, breathe, and gather strength for the prolonged intimacy of vigil hours. Its positioning by the window creates a dual relationship: The watcher maintains closeness to the patient while simultaneously encountering the world outside, grounding themselves through sky, trees, shifting light, or distant movement. This gentle connection to the natural world provides solace, perspective, and temporal orientation during moments when internal time may feel disjointed or suspended.

Ergonomics and comfort are crucial, as vigil hours often stretch into long, uninterrupted sequences. Upholstery must be soft yet supportive, enabling hours of sitting without strain on the back, neck, or hips. High backs, gentle recline, and cushioned armrests allow watchers to maintain comfortable posture, and materials such as wool, linen, and soft leather create tactile warmth and encourage physical endurance. Attention to such details allows caregivers and family members to remain physically present without distraction, supporting emotional engagement and sustaining the quiet companionship that often defines end-of-life moments.

Stories abound of families spending entire nights in vigil chairs, observing breath patterns, holding hands, or whispering reassurances as they accompany loved ones through their final hours. These chairs bear witness to some of the most intimate human experiences: vulnerability, love, grief, and the slow rhythms of dying. One family recalled watching dawn rise through the window as they sat in the vigil chairs, tracking the patient's chest rise and fall with each shift in natural light. That morning became a marker—not only of time passing but also of life transitioning into memory. Such narratives reveal how the chair becomes a vessel for emotional endurance, relational devotion, and the silent rituals of farewell.

The placement by the window serves multiple intertwined functions. Natural light, shifting gradually throughout the day, offers temporal orientation and a sense of continuity, helping family members track the passage of hours without reliance on clocks or external cues. Glimpses of sky, birds, trees, or distant activity connect the room to a larger world, reminding both the watcher and the patient that life persists beyond the room's emotional intensity. The window also provides symbolic framing: life moving outward, continuing, evolving, even as attention remains focused inward on the precious intimacy of the moment.

The chair becomes a metaphor for witnessing both life and letting go. Sitting vigil is, by its very nature, a liminal experience—one that bridges presence and acceptance, attention and surrender. By positioning the chair near a window, hospice design allows watchers to hold two realities at once: the internal world of imminent loss and the external world of continuity, movement, and change. This delicate tension finds physical expression in the chair's placement, giving form to the emotional balancing act of remaining close while preparing to release.

Ergonomic design extends beyond the chair itself to include foot support, flexibility, and adaptability. Reclining options, small ottomans, or adjustable footrests allow watchers to shift posture, reducing physical strain during long periods of stillness. These features may seem modest, but they support endurance and make sustained presence possible, ensuring that physical discomfort does not pull attention away from emotional connection. In this way, the chair becomes an enabler of relational attention rather than a mere piece of furniture.

The visual presence of the chair communicates relational priority to anyone entering the room. When positioned intentionally—angled toward the bed, but open enough to the window to support reflective gaze—it signals that the room is a site of attention, care, and companionship. Families instinctively orient themselves toward it, forming behavioral patterns that respect the patient's dignity while allowing for structured observation and relational closeness. Its very placement becomes a quiet architectural cue that tenderness belongs here.

The tactile quality of upholstery also matters profoundly, particularly in moments when touch becomes a primary means of connection. Fabrics that are warm, soft, and slightly textured invite extended contact—hands resting on armrests, fingers brushing fabric while leaning forward, or steadying oneself during an emotional swell. These tactile experiences enhance emotional resonance and reinforce relational continuity, offering comfort not only through physical support but also through sensory grounding during the vigil.

Lighting near the chair is carefully considered to avoid harshness while providing enough visibility for reading, reflection, or gentle nighttime wakefulness. Soft, adjustable lamps or filtered natural light from the window creates a serene environment conducive to contemplation and quiet presence. By illuminating the vigil spot without disturbing the patient, this lighting supports equilibrium in the room, balancing necessary clarity with emotional calm and ensuring that the watcher can remain grounded without overwhelming the space.

The chair also serves as a stage for ritualized actions that become part of the vigil's emotional choreography. Whether placing a hand gently over the patient's, adjusting a blanket, reading aloud, or offering whispered affirmations, the watcher performs these gestures from a dedicated spot that lends structure to their movements. The physical boundary of the chair creates a psychological container, helping watchers understand their role, their proximity, and their capacity for care within the room.

Stories of vigil emphasize relational continuity and the long arc of human connection. A daughter sitting for hours recounting childhood memories, a spouse whispering decades-old promises, and a sibling holding a patient's hand while watching the daylight fade all highlight the chair as an anchor for enduring presence. These intimate stories illustrate how the chair mediates emotional, spatial, and relational dynamics, enabling watchers to remain steady, attentive, and present without becoming overwhelmed.

Positioning relative to the patient is critical, ensuring that the watcher can maintain unobstructed sightlines while preserving a sense of personal space. When placed properly, the chair supports sustained engagement without creating the impression of intrusion or surveillance. It allows watchers to maintain attention in a way that feels natural, warm, and respectful, supporting psychological safety for both patient and family.

Windows provide a subtle cue for circadian orientation, which is particularly important during extended vigils when internal time can blur. Shifts in natural light—dawn brightening, afternoon warming, dusk softening—communicate the rhythm of the day and help maintain orientation for both the patient and family. For patients in their final hours, aligning with natural cues may reduce disorientation; for families, these cues create a temporal narrative that frames the vigil within the larger unfolding of time.

The chair embodies both stability and adaptability. It must remain sturdy to ensure safety and support, yet it must be flexible enough to accommodate multiple family members, cultural practices, or rituals of care. Features such as swivel, recline, and adjustable arm height allow the chair to serve diverse purposes, all while maintaining its central role as a locus of witness, reflection, and presence. The combination of solidity and flexibility mirrors the emotional dynamics of vigil itself.

Materials age in ways that reinforce emotional resonance. A well-used vigil chair absorbs subtle traces of presence over time—softened upholstery, worn armrests, slight depressions in the seat—creating a sense of history and continuity. Families often remark on the "comforting familiarity" of a chair that seems to have held countless watchers before them, linking their experience to a lineage of care that extends far beyond the present moment.

The psychological benefit of a dedicated vigil spot cannot be overstated. Families consistently report that having a defined place to sit reduces anxiety, structures their presence, and provides a safe container for experiencing the intensity of watching. The chair's role is not only physical but also emotional: it grants permission to be still, to remain present, to breathe, and to process the unfolding moment without feeling compelled to act constantly or move around the room.

Even after death, the chair retains its symbolic significance. It stands as a witness, a silent participant in the rituals of goodbye, memory, and reflection. Families often pause near the chair in final moments, acknowledging the support it provided and the emotional labor it held. In these moments, the chair becomes a physical marker of relational continuity, embodying the care, devotion, and presence that defined the vigil.

The window chair integrates spatial, psychological, and symbolic considerations, uniting them into a single architectural expression of care. It aligns ergonomic comfort with visual engagement, connects interior space with the natural world, supports ritualized behavior, and mediates the emotional intensity of vigil. In doing so, it exemplifies the larger truth that hospice architecture and furniture serve not only functional purposes but also deeply human and emotional ones, shaping how we remain present during the most profound transitions of life.

Textiles and fabrics within a hospice room serve purposes far beyond physical comfort or aesthetic appeal. Blankets, quilts, sheets, and pillows become carriers of memory, symbols of care, and tools of emotional regulation. A blanket brought from home can evoke the scent, warmth, and familiarity of the patient's daily life, bridging the gap between the intimate world they have known and the unfamiliarity of a clinical environment. Such fabrics carry personal and familial histories, anchoring identity and memory while offering reassurance during moments of vulnerability.[4]

Weighted blankets, increasingly incorporated into hospice care, serve not only a functional role in temperature regulation but also as sensory tools for emotional stabilization. The gentle pressure of a weighted blanket can soothe agitation, anxiety, or terminal restlessness, supporting both physical and psychological calm. This type of tactile input interacts with the autonomic nervous system, fostering a sense of security and grounding that is particularly valuable in end-of-life care. By integrating weighted textiles, caregivers create nonpharmacologic pathways to comfort that supplement medical interventions.

Bed linens themselves convey a profound psychological message. Hospital-grade sheets and sterile bedding often reinforce clinical, impersonal atmospheres. Replacing them with soft cotton, linen, or flannel sheets that echo home environments immediately signals warmth, familiarity, and relational care. Families often describe how this subtle shift transforms the patient's room into a safe, emotionally resonant space, encouraging both patients and loved ones to relax and be present without the anxiety-inducing cues of institutional sterility.

Cultural textile practices add layers of meaning and ritual to hospice care. In Jewish tradition, a prayer shawl may be draped over or near the patient during specific moments. In Catholic care, small sacred cloths or altar cloths may accompany bedside prayers. Indigenous and other cultural traditions often use handmade quilts, ceremonial fabrics, or woven items as both protective and symbolic tools. Incorporating culturally significant textiles into hospice design not only honors spiritual practices but also reinforces family participation in meaningful ritualized care.[5]

Texture plays a central role in relational behavior and emotional connection. Soft, inviting fabrics encourage physical closeness, such as leaning over the bed, holding hands, or resting a cheek on a pillow. Tactile engagement strengthens relational presence, provides comfort, and fosters prolonged attention during vigil hours. The interplay between touch, memory, and emotional regulation underscores the significance of fabrics in shaping both the psychological and relational dimensions of hospice care.

Bringing textiles from home is often a deliberate act of symbolic care. Families select blankets, quilts, or pillows that carry personal histories—whether associated with travel, holidays, or other shared memories. By introducing these objects into the hospice room, families embed narrative, identity, and love into the physical environment, creating a layered emotional landscape that extends beyond immediate comfort into the realm of memory preservation and relational presence.

Staff often integrate these comfort textiles into care routines intentionally. Draping a familiar blanket, adjusting the folds of a quilt, or replacing clinical linens with home-like sheets communicates attentiveness and empathy. Such acts reinforce dignity, reduce anxiety, and demonstrate relational care. The interaction between staff and family in arranging textiles also supports shared participation in the emotional environment, fostering trust and continuity in care.

Weighted and specialty fabrics provide additional support for both patient and family. When a patient's restlessness is reduced, families are able to remain present longer and participate more fully in vigil, observation, and shared reflection. The textiles, therefore, serve not only as comfort devices for the patient but also as facilitators of relational engagement, sustaining emotional attention during critical hours.

The layering of textiles contributes both functionally and symbolically. A base sheet, a quilt, a throw, and an optional weighted blanket can each convey a different type of care, providing multiple levels of tactile, visual, and emotional comfort. Families often engage with these layers by adjusting, smoothing, or repositioning them during vigils, reinforcing ritualized patterns of behavior while maintaining patient comfort and dignity.

Color and pattern choices in hospice textiles also impact the emotional tone of the room. Muted and soothing colors foster calm and reflection, whereas patterns that carry personal or familial significance can evoke familiarity and relational connection. Thoughtful coordination between textiles, lighting, and furniture ensures that the room's visual cues align with its emotional intent, creating a cohesive sensory and symbolic environment.

Memory and legacy are embedded in textiles. Quilts passed down through generations, blankets handmade by loved ones, or fabrics associated with significant events all serve as tangible carriers of identity. The tactile engagement with these items allows both patient and family to reconnect with meaningful stories and shared histories, reinforcing the emotional narrative of care.

Textiles also accommodate spiritual and ritual practices. Prayer shawls, altar cloths, or ceremonial fabrics enable families to perform faith-based rituals directly in the patient's environment. Strategic placement ensures visibility and accessibility, facilitating ritualized gestures that align with personal or cultural traditions while maintaining room functionality.

The tactile interaction with fabrics enhances emotional resonance. Simple gestures, such as adjusting a blanket, stroking a quilt, or holding a pillow while whispering to the patient, allow family members to communicate care nonverbally. These interactions become part of the ritualized acts of presence that define hospice care, providing a channel for emotional expression when words are insufficient.

Textile durability and care are important practical considerations. Fabrics must withstand frequent handling, laundering, and long-term use while maintaining softness and warmth. Attention to material selection ensures that these items remain effective as comfort objects over time, supporting both physical and emotional functions without loss of sensory or symbolic value.

Memory textiles can also structure the room spatially. Draping a quilt over a vigil chair, folding a blanket on the bedside table, or arranging throws at accessible points establishes zones of attention, reflection, and relational focus. These cues subtly guide behavior, shaping how families interact with the patient and the environment during vigil periods.

Families frequently incorporate textiles into rituals. Covering the patient with a specific quilt during a prayer, smoothing a blanket during silent reflection, or placing a favorite throw over the lap transforms ordinary actions into symbolic gestures. These rituals, mediated through fabric, help organize time, attention, and relational behavior during the emotional intensity of hospice care.

The interplay of textiles and light reinforces their effect. Soft fabrics reflect warm illumination, contributing to a visually and emotionally comforting environment. During twilight or night hours, the combination of gentle light and tactile comfort creates a sacred, contemplative atmosphere conducive to vigil, reflection, and relational engagement.

Textiles also function as transitional objects after death. Leaving a blanket or quilt momentarily in place allows family members to maintain continuity with the patient's presence, providing a tangible focus during the early stages of grief. These objects serve as both memory anchors and instruments of comfort, supporting emotional processing and relational continuity.

Ultimately, comfort textiles illustrate the broader principle of hospice design: Small, personal, and tactile objects can profoundly mediate emotional, psychological, and relational experiences. Through texture, familiarity, ritual, and memory, fabrics transform a clinical room into an emotionally and spiritually resonant environment, supporting presence, care, and the human dimensions of the dying process.

Time in the hospice room is both present and elusive. The simple presence of a clock can evoke comfort, anxiety, or reflection, depending on its design, placement, and the psychological state of those in the room. The ticking of a clock can mark the rhythm of life, reminding family members of the passage of moments, or it can feel oppressive, amplifying awareness of mortality. Understanding these nuances is central to designing spaces that honor both emotional and temporal needs.

Different philosophies guide whether a ticking clock should be present in a hospice room. Some caregivers find that a subtle auditory rhythm provides reassurance and structure, a gentle pulse against the uncertainty of dying. Others argue that even a soft tick heightens anxiety, magnifying the sense of impending loss. Decisions about clock presence, sound, and placement should always be made with sensitivity to the family's and patient's preferences, creating a room that supports emotional equilibrium.

Time perception shifts profoundly in the dying room. Minutes can stretch into what feels like hours, and hours may dissolve into timelessness. Families often describe vigil hours as simultaneously long and fleeting, as though temporal markers are suspended. This altered perception is part of the emotional intensity of hospice care, underscoring the need for both literal and symbolic tools to mediate the experience of passing time.

Some hospice rooms intentionally silence clocks to reduce sensory distraction and create an impression of temporal fluidity. Without the auditory cue of ticking, families and caregivers report feeling more attuned to the subtle rhythms of breathing, pulse, and movement, heightening relational presence. This silence allows the room itself to set the pace, governed by the interaction of people, rituals, and light rather than mechanical measurement.

The ritual of removing the clock battery after death is a profound gesture, marking closure and the cessation of measured time. This small act transforms an ordinary object into a symbolic participant in the dying process. It communicates both respect and acknowledgment that the patient has transcended the constraints of chronological time, and it signals to family members that the structured measurement of minutes is no longer necessary in the room.

Horology, the study and measurement of time, carries metaphorical significance in hospice care. Clocks serve as companions, quietly witnessing the unfolding of final hours. They bear silent testimony to the shared presence of families, caregivers, and patients, transforming ordinary objects into narrative devices that mark human attention, devotion, and endurance.

The clock can also embody the notion of time as witness. Just as a photograph preserves a visual moment, the presence of a clock during vigil hours captures the intangible rhythm of care. The gentle advance of the hands, or the subtle marking of the second, becomes part of the spatial memory of the room, embedding temporal continuity into the emotional landscape.

Placement of the clock within the room affects perception and function. A clock positioned directly above the patient may amplify anxiety, whereas one placed peripherally, partially obscured, or with muted design allows families to orient themselves without constant awareness of minutes. Design choices around size, sound, and placement subtly influence how time is experienced and internalized.

Families often describe the experience of vigil as being "outside" conventional time. Hours of quiet observation, punctuated by small gestures of care or whispered conversation, feel both infinite and fleeting. In these moments, the clock functions less as a practical tool and more as a symbolic companion, affirming presence while acknowledging the irrelevance of measured minutes.

The clock's visual design communicates meaning as well. Minimalist faces, soft contrasts, and absence of loud ticking create calm, whereas overly clinical or decorative clocks may impose unintended emotional tone. Designers must consider aesthetic, auditory, and symbolic aspects when integrating clocks into hospice rooms, ensuring that the object aligns with the room's emotional and psychological purpose.

Some cultures and faith traditions imbue timekeeping objects with spiritual significance. In certain Buddhist practices, the marking of temporal intervals can serve as cues for meditation or prayer, whereas in Christian settings, subtle reference to time may reflect divine ordering. Integrating culturally resonant timepieces into hospice design reinforces ritualized care and provides tangible cues that align with familial and spiritual values.

The removal of the clock battery after death has practical, symbolic, and emotional dimensions. Practically, it silences mechanical measurement, preventing distraction. Symbolically, it marks the finality of passage. Emotionally, it allows family members to shift focus from chronological tracking to memory, reflection, and grief, framing the room as a site of relational and temporal transcendence.

Even small timepieces, such as bedside watches or tabletop clocks, contribute to the room's layered narrative. Their presence, absence, or placement mediates engagement with time, subtly shaping attention, movement, and ritual behavior. The careful curation of these objects aligns functional, aesthetic, and emotional priorities in hospice design.

Family members often ascribe narrative qualities to the clock. Watching the second hand move, noting the slow passing of minutes, or witnessing dawn through a window aligned with the clock can create temporal markers that support storytelling, reflection, and continuity. The clock becomes a subtle narrator of presence and attention, integrating ordinary objects into the emotional landscape of care.

Time in hospice is simultaneously linear and relational. Clocks measure linear intervals, but relational time—how long a family member sits, how long a nurse observes, how long a vigil lasts—is qualitatively different. Hospice design acknowledges this duality, ensuring that clocks neither dominate the emotional experience nor become irrelevant, but instead function as flexible mediators of presence.

Some rooms incorporate soft, natural cues to complement or replace clocks: shifting daylight, filtered sunlight, or subtle lighting changes. These cues create a temporal rhythm grounded in natural phenomena rather than mechanical measurement, helping families and patients attune to the passage of time in a more organic, less clinical manner.

The clock also functions as a mnemonic device. Its silent or ticking presence anchors memory of vigil, prayer, or shared reflection. Families often recall "the hour the sun fell on the hands of the clock" or "the minute the battery was removed" as markers that integrate physical and emotional memory. In this sense, clocks become storytellers, embedding moments of relational attention into the room's narrative.

Designers sometimes offer the choice between analog and digital clocks. Analog clocks, with sweeping hands, communicate continuous passage and rhythm, whereas digital displays may feel abrupt or mechanical. Choice of display is not purely aesthetic; it impacts emotional perception, cognitive load, and family comfort, reinforcing the need for intentional design decisions.

The relationship between light and clock perception is critical. Clocks illuminated by soft, indirect light support gentle awareness of time without drawing attention away from relational presence. Harsh illumination or prominent positioning may interfere with vigil focus or induce stress. Lighting and clock design must thus be harmonized to support emotional and spatial coherence.

Finally, the hospice clock functions as the room's last storyteller. Beyond marking minutes, it communicates witness, presence, and continuity. It mediates attention, structures ritual, and provides a symbolic framework for understanding the passage of life and the transition into memory. In this way, even the simplest clock embodies complex emotional, cultural, and psychological significance, confirming that every object in a hospice room participates in the narrative of care, attention, and remembrance.

4
Rituals of Comfort and Continuity

The micro-rituals of daily hospice care form the invisible architecture of presence, structure, and dignity. In a room designed for emotional attunement, these rituals carry a weight far beyond their practical function. Each small action—the touch of a washcloth, the brushing of hair, the offering of water—acts as both care and communication. They are the subtle language of attentiveness, signaling that the patient is valued, seen, and honored.

The warm washcloth ritual exemplifies this dual role of care and symbolic gesture. Gently warming a cloth in water and placing it over the patient's hands or face communicates attention, tenderness, and respect. The warmth and moisture provide sensory grounding, offering a momentary relief from discomfort, while the careful handling conveys nonverbal reassurance. This ritual, repeated daily, forms a predictable cadence, comforting both patient and family members.[1]

Hair brushing is another seemingly simple gesture with profound emotional resonance. At the bedside, running a soft brush through the patient's hair restores a sense of identity and selfhood. For patients who feel disoriented or fatigued, this action reconnects them to their own body, their sense of grooming and appearance, and often evokes memory of personal routines from earlier life stages. Families witnessing this ritual often feel reassured, perceiving continuity and care in the patient's embodied presence.

Hydration rituals, such as offering water through a small cup, spoon, or straw, blend practical necessity with symbolic care. A sip of water represents attentiveness and nurturance. The caregiver's slow, careful approach communicates a deep relational presence, allowing patients to experience care as relationally intimate rather than purely functional. Water becomes both sustenance and a medium for communication, a way to affirm life even in the final hours.

Soft voice protocols are essential in these rituals. Staff modulate tone, pace, and cadence during vigil hours to create an atmosphere of calm, reassurance, and relational focus. The gentle murmur of a caregiver's voice, timed with breathing or movement, fosters trust and emotional attunement. Families often adopt similar vocal patterns, learning from staff how to interact without overwhelming or startling the patient. Voice modulation thus becomes a ritualized skill that structures presence as much as any physical action.[2]

These micro-rituals create a rhythm within the room that families learn to anticipate. Regular timing of washcloth application, hair care, or hydration visits forms temporal markers, helping relatives structure their own presence. Even small gestures—adjusting a blanket, smoothing a pillow, or repositioning a chair—acquire ritual significance, forming a collective choreography that underscores care, attention, and continuity.

The tactile dimension of these rituals is particularly important. The sense of touch conveys information, reassurance, and connection in ways words cannot. The warmth of a washcloth, the pressure of a brush through hair, or the gentle placement of a hand during hydration communicates attentiveness and empathy, reinforcing relational bonds. For patients nearing the end of life, tactile contact becomes a central mode of perceiving care.

Micro-rituals also structure emotional experience. They provide predictable, comforting sequences that families can learn and replicate. This predictability reduces anxiety, offers a sense of control, and enables meaningful participation in the patient's care. Families often describe feeling "anchored" by these repeated acts, knowing that their attention and love are materially expressed and mirrored in ritualized behavior.

Even the smallest gestures carry symbolic meaning. Adjusting a blanket or smoothing a sheet communicates protection, attentiveness, and relational presence. These actions may appear mundane to an outside observer, but within the emotional and temporal context of hospice, they acquire profound significance.

The sequencing of rituals matters. Caregivers often follow established micro-routines: washing hands, offering water, adjusting linens, brushing hair, and then pausing for reflection or quiet. This sequence becomes both functional and symbolic, signaling transitions between care activities while creating a narrative flow for the day. Families can enter this rhythm, observing, assisting, or simply being present during each step.

Rituals also modulate emotional intensity in the room. Gentle gestures, repeated actions, and predictable routines provide a counterbalance to the heightened anxiety or grief that can accompany hospice care. In this way, micro-rituals serve as emotional regulators, stabilizing both patients and families through their consistency and attentional focus.

These gestures are not merely mechanical but deeply relational. The intention behind each action communicates care, respect, and emotional attunement. Families often report that observing or participating in these rituals provides comfort, reassurance, and a sense of shared purpose, reinforcing both connection and continuity.

Micro-rituals create a shared language between staff, patients, and family members. The gentle application of a warm cloth, the brushing of hair, or the offering of water becomes an unspoken communication, a bridge between those performing care and those receiving it. This shared language fosters intimacy, mutual understanding, and emotional resonance.

The aesthetic quality of the room enhances these rituals. Soft lighting, minimal clutter, and thoughtful material choices create a sensory backdrop that supports ritualized behaviors. Families and staff respond more readily to subtle gestures in environments in which sensory stressors are minimized, reinforcing the importance of architectural design in shaping care.

Time perception is intimately linked to ritual. The repetition of small gestures slows subjective experience, providing space for reflection, presence, and attentiveness. Families often note that hours spent in vigil seem both extended and compressed: Rituals create temporal anchors that help participants navigate the elasticity of time during end-of-life care.

Micro-rituals serve as scaffolding for grief. Participating in these gestures allows family members to express care, presence, and love tangibly, providing a sense of agency when other aspects of the dying process feel uncontrollable. These acts of attention become enduring memories, anchoring the experience of caregiving in concrete, relational behavior.

Even the silent rituals—the repositioning of a hand, the smoothing of a blanket, the subtle adjustment of a pillow—convey presence. These understated gestures reinforce relational bonds and emotional attunement, demonstrating that care is conveyed as much through action as through speech.

Cultural adaptations of micro-rituals further enrich the hospice experience. Families may integrate religious or spiritual elements, such as blessings, prayers, or symbolic gestures, into routines of washing, brushing, or offering water. These adaptations honor individual belief systems and enhance the meaningfulness of everyday acts of care.[3]

The durability of ritual is evident over time. Families returning to participate in vigil repeatedly engage with the same set of micro-actions, reinforcing continuity and relational presence. Rituals accumulate meaning with repetition, transforming ordinary caregiving activities into sacred acts of attention, love, and witnessing.

Finally, the micro-rituals of daily hospice care illustrate the profound intersection of architecture, objects, and human behavior. Even the smallest gestures—guided by intention, environmental design, and relational presence—create a framework for dignity, emotional attunement, and continuity. These rituals, repeated and observed over time, form the heartbeat of hospice care, embedding relational and emotional memory within both the space and the lived experience of those present.

Family rituals in hospice care represent the tangible expression of love, memory, and presence. These small, deliberate acts allow relatives to participate actively in the caregiving process, bridging the emotional distance that can emerge as death approaches. The rituals are both practical and symbolic, providing structure, comfort, and a shared language of presence that strengthens relational bonds.

Repositioning the blanket is one of the simplest yet most profound family rituals. Adjusting the folds, smoothing wrinkles, or tucking the fabric gently communicates care and attention. When done collectively, family members participate in the act as a shared gesture of devotion. This minor yet deliberate involvement conveys love, sustains dignity, and allows relatives to physically inhabit the caregiving process alongside staff, reinforcing continuity of presence.

Night-watch rituals emerge naturally during the vigil. Families often maintain journals, whisper stories from the patient's life, or read aloud favorite poems or letters. These activities structure time during long, quiet hours, providing meaning and relational continuity. The act of storytelling affirms the patient's identity and legacy, allowing narratives to unfold while reinforcing emotional closeness.

Hand-holding circles are another powerful ritual. Family members often form a ring around the patient, physically linking hands or resting fingers on arms and shoulders. This configuration communicates collective support, protection, and shared witness. The circle becomes a symbolic container for presence, grief, and love, stabilizing the emotional environment and giving everyone a role in attending to the dying person.

Cultural family rituals shape these experiences in unique ways. Singing, prayer, recitation, incense, or periods of silence are often integrated into the room's rhythm. Families draw upon personal belief systems to infuse the environment with meaning, offering the patient spiritual comfort and reinforcing the continuity of cultural identity. Staff facilitate these practices by ensuring that space, lighting, and objects accommodate them without disruption.

"Permission rituals" help family members voice acceptance and encourage the patient to let go. Phrases such as "It's alright to rest now," whispered or accompanied by touch, provide a structured, socially sanctioned means for expressing release and emotional surrender. These rituals ease tension, help manage anticipatory grief, and create psychological space for transition, supporting both the patient and loved ones.

The placement of chairs, blankets, and other objects during family rituals is intentionally choreographed. Families often cluster around the bed, placing personal objects or photographs within reach. This spatial arrangement reinforces engagement, provides tactile anchors, and encourages participation in micro-gestures of care. The room itself thus becomes a stage for ritualized interaction, enabling relational presence to unfold naturally.

Families frequently adapt micro-rituals into extended sequences. Adjusting linens, offering water, holding hands, and sharing stories may be repeated in cycles, creating predictable rhythms that reduce anxiety and help participants manage emotional intensity. These sequences provide temporal markers, structuring otherwise amorphous hours and allowing families to navigate both presence and absence meaningfully.

Lighting and sound cues support family rituals. Soft illumination focuses attention on the patient while minimizing environmental distraction. Gentle background sounds—filtered music, the whisper of the nurse, or the muted hum of the room—reinforce intimacy without intruding on ritualized behavior. These sensory cues act as subtle signals for timing and pacing, guiding participation without overt instruction.

Objects serve as focal points during family rituals. Photographs, religious symbols, personal mementos, or a cherished blanket provide visual and tactile anchors. These items encourage storytelling, reminiscence, and attentional focus, allowing relatives to interact relationally with both the patient and the memory of their shared life. Objects become mediums for continuity, memory, and emotional expression.

Storytelling rituals often incorporate humor, reflection, or reminiscence. Families recount events from childhood, achievements, or shared experiences, embedding laughter and tears within the vigil hours. These narratives help patients feel remembered and valued, while relatives process grief through relational and narrative engagement. The act of telling reinforces the continuity of identity beyond the immediate dying process.

Silence itself becomes a ritual. Families may observe quiet intervals, allowing presence to speak for itself. In these moments, attention is conveyed through posture, touch, and gaze, emphasizing relational attunement. Silence provides a container for reflection, prayer, or meditation, and it allows the patient's presence to be fully witnessed without the interference of speech or external noise.

The timing of rituals often coincides with natural environmental markers. Dawn, sunset, or the transition from day to night can trigger specific practices, such as reading, recitation, or symbolic gestures. These temporal cues link the patient's experience to natural rhythms, reinforcing continuity and providing a framework for emotional engagement.

Family rituals often evolve organically. Initially hesitant or unsure, relatives gradually assume roles and actions that feel appropriate within the room's relational context. Staff guidance is crucial in these early stages, helping families identify meaningful gestures, understand their emotional significance, and recognize the shared purpose of the ritual.

Physical touch is central to many rituals. Holding a hand, brushing hair, smoothing a blanket, or gently stroking a shoulder communicates presence, reassurance, and love. These acts provide both patient and family with sensory confirmation of care and relational connection, reinforcing dignity and mitigating fear or disorientation.

Ritualized storytelling often incorporates shared reading or journaling. Family members write notes, recall memories, or read aloud reflections, creating temporal and emotional markers that structure vigil hours. These written or spoken narratives function as both present engagement and enduring memory, forming an intergenerational record of care and presence.

Song and music rituals are also common. Singing familiar hymns, spiritual chants, or songs with personal significance can soothe anxiety, reinforce cultural identity, and create an auditory landscape conducive to reflection and attention. Music provides rhythm, emotional resonance, and a shared sensory experience that strengthens relational bonds.

The integration of ritual objects, sound, touch, and light creates a multisensory environment that amplifies emotional resonance. These elements converge to form a coherent, layered experience in which care, presence, and love are expressed in complementary modalities. The design of the room, therefore, directly influences the effectiveness and emotional impact of family rituals.

Rituals also facilitate anticipatory grief processing. By actively participating in gestures of care, family members acknowledge the impending loss while expressing ongoing love and attention. These actions provide psychological scaffolding, allowing relatives to move between hope, acceptance, and emotional preparation in a structured and meaningful manner.

Even post-death, family rituals maintain significance. Leaving objects in place, repeating gestures of touch, or reciting familiar phrases can help relatives bridge the transition from active caregiving to remembrance. These ongoing practices reinforce the continuity of memory and relational presence, confirming that rituals extend beyond life into enduring emotional landscapes.

Ultimately, family rituals in hospice care exemplify the profound interplay between physical space, objects, relational attention, and emotional support. Each gesture—whether repositioning a blanket, holding a hand, sharing a story, or observing silence—creates patterns of love, continuity, and witness that define the emotional architecture of the final days.

Staff rituals in hospice are subtle yet profoundly shaping forces within the care environment. Unlike the visible family rituals, these practices are often unspoken, internalized through experience, and enacted with both precision and empathy. They provide structure, continuity, and emotional calibration for professionals who witness the cyclical intensity of life and death on a daily basis.

One of the most emblematic staff rituals is the pause following a patient's passing. Nurses, aides, and chaplains often take a deliberate moment of silence, allowing themselves to register the transition before beginning any practical tasks. This pause honors the individual, acknowledges the relational depth of the care provided, and reinforces professional presence in the moment of ultimate vulnerability. It is a ritualized acknowledgment that life's passage merits reflection, not only action.

The room-reset ritual is another central practice. After the patient has passed, staff meticulously smooth blankets, straighten pillows, close curtains, and tidy bedside surfaces. Each gesture is carried out with reverence, as if preparing the space to preserve the dignity of the deceased. These acts serve dual functions: They restore the room's physical order while symbolically signaling closure and respect. The careful arrangement of space communicates to both family and staff that the transition has been honored.

Spiritual care rituals are frequently embedded in staff practices. Chaplains, for example, may place a small stone, a flower, or a card with a blessing on the bedside table. These gestures are often quietly performed, without fanfare, yet carry enormous symbolic weight. They reinforce the notion that death is not solely a clinical event but also a deeply human and spiritual moment, acknowledging the patient's and family's values and beliefs.

Debriefing rituals among staff are vital for emotional processing. After particularly challenging or poignant deaths, teams gather to reflect, share observations, and support each other. This practice is both practical and symbolic: It maintains professional cohesion, mitigates burnout, and fosters emotional resilience by validating the shared experience of care. These debriefings also reinforce professional identity, reminding staff of their purpose and the meaningful impact of their work.

Staff rituals extend beyond these highly visible gestures. Daily micro-actions—checking comfort measures, adjusting lighting, softening tones of voice, and maintaining an unobtrusive presence—constitute a continuous practice of attunement. Each action, while seemingly mundane, is embedded in an ethos of care and respect, reinforcing the emotional and physical architecture of the hospice room.

The pause, the room reset, and other staff rituals contribute to the creation of sacred space within the hospice environment. They signal transitions, mark the passage of life, and structure relational dynamics in ways that are emotionally intelligible to both families and staff. These rituals create a rhythm that mirrors natural cycles of attention, caregiving, and closure, reinforcing both human and environmental continuity.

Ritualized cleaning and arrangement of objects carry psychological significance. By methodically tending to the room, staff externalize respect, transforming practical tasks into gestures of moral and emotional care. The tactile and visual reordering of the environment becomes a medium through which grief, acknowledgment, and presence are expressed without words.

The integration of spiritual artifacts—stones, flowers, or cards—serves as a tangible extension of ritualized care. These objects act as symbols of witness, memory, and blessing, anchoring the room with quiet intentionality. Their placement is deliberate, often corresponding to the spatial geometry of the room and the patient's position, ensuring that each gesture communicates both reverence and relational attunement.

Staff also ritualize transitions within the day. Morning rounds, shift changes, and evening vigils often include structured sequences: lighting adjustments, environmental checks, and informal consultations among team members. These repeated actions structure temporal awareness, signaling care continuity and emotional stability for patients and families alike.

In addition, ritualized gestures mediate emotional intensity. By incorporating brief pauses, deliberate touches, or quiet acknowledgments, staff can regulate their own emotional responses and those of families. These actions are subtle yet critical, providing psychological containment during periods of heightened vulnerability.

Observation is a ritual in itself. Staff develop an unspoken attentiveness to micro-expressions, subtle breathing patterns, and small environmental cues. These acts of careful noticing allow for timely intervention, emotional support, and adaptive care, reflecting a deep interplay between human perception and professional ritualization.

Staff rituals foster relational continuity, both among team members and with patients and families. By adhering to established patterns of behavior—such as standardized room resets, ceremonial pauses, and ritualized spiritual acts—professionals create a shared understanding of presence, care, and respect that transcends individual staff members' shifts or roles.

The symbolic language of staff rituals often parallels family rituals. For example, smoothing blankets or adjusting a pillow may mirror a family member's gesture, creating synchronicity and reinforcing collective witness. This mirroring strengthens relational and emotional coherence, demonstrating how ritual serves as a bridge between professional and familial care.

Debriefing sessions often include reflective storytelling. Staff recount moments of connection, humor, or insight observed during care. These narrative practices are themselves ritualized, helping teams process complex emotions, reinforce professional identity, and sustain empathy across successive patient encounters.

Rituals also provide emotional resilience. The repeated enactment of small, meaningful gestures cultivates a sense of mastery, intentionality, and moral coherence. This consistency helps staff navigate the unpredictability of death, providing psychological scaffolding that supports ongoing compassion and presence.

Spatial awareness is integral to staff rituals. Movement through the room—approaching the bedside, adjusting lighting, or handling objects—is choreographed to minimize disruption and maximize emotional and relational impact. Staff develop intuitive knowledge of these micro-pathways, enhancing the efficacy of rituals and reinforcing the room's emotional architecture.

The layering of auditory, tactile, and visual rituals amplifies their effect. Soft-spoken words, gentle handling of fabrics, and careful placement of objects coalesce into a coherent sensory narrative that structures both attention and emotional response. These elements converge to create a ritualized environment that communicates care beyond verbal language.

Staff rituals also function as tacit teaching tools. Junior team members learn through observation, imitation, and guided participation, internalizing the unspoken codes of presence, respect, and relational attention. This ritualized apprenticeship ensures continuity of practice and preserves the emotional intelligence embedded in hospice care.

Finally, staff rituals affirm the moral and professional ethos of hospice. Through intentional pauses, reverent handling of space, spiritual gestures, and debriefing, professionals maintain integrity, sustain emotional health, and enact care that honors both patient and family. These rituals transform the hospice room into a space of relational, emotional, and symbolic significance, ensuring that every act of attention contributes to the enduring narrative of love, witness, and closure.

Cultural and spiritual rituals are essential elements of hospice care, shaping the emotional, sensory, and symbolic experience of patients and families. Designing spaces that honor these rituals requires careful attention to architecture, objects, sound, light, and circulation, creating an environment in which multiple traditions can coexist without conflict or hierarchy.

Flame-free candle alternatives exemplify the intersection of ritual and safety. LED candles or fiber-optic "flames" provide the flickering, warm light desired in many cultural ceremonies while eliminating fire hazards. This design choice allows families to maintain symbolic acts such as lighting a candle at the bedside, creating sacred time, or marking transitions without compromising the safety protocols of a clinical setting.

Adjustable ventilation and air control are equally important. Certain rituals, such as smudging, incense burning, or aromatic offerings, require airflow management. By integrating discreet ventilation systems, architects ensure that the sensory environment remains comfortable, odor levels are controlled, and rituals can be enacted without impacting other patients or staff. Movable partitions or furniture allow flexibility, accommodating both private and semipublic ceremonial arrangements.

Bed placement can honor directional significance in religious traditions. For example, some Hindu, Buddhist, or Indigenous practices emphasize specific orientations—such as facing east for rebirth or north for ancestral connection.

Thoughtful positioning of the patient bed, chairs, and ritual objects can respect these requirements, demonstrating cultural attunement while preserving functional and aesthetic flow.

Music rituals are another critical component of cultural and spiritual care. Drums, chanting, hymns, throat singing, or curated spiritual playlists support the emotional and spiritual needs of the patient. Rooms designed with subtle acoustical treatments, low-frequency absorption, and speaker placement allow these rituals to resonate without disturbing adjacent areas. Music becomes a medium for memory, attention, and presence, reinforcing the sanctity of end-of-life moments.

Ritual objects play a central role in cultural observance. Rosaries, prayer blankets, malas, symbolic stones, smudge kits, scripture books, or other items provide tactile and visual anchors for spiritual engagement. Storage and display systems—open shelves, small altars, or dedicated alcoves—allow objects to be accessible, visible, and organized without creating clutter. This spatial integration elevates the objects from mere decoration to active participants in ritualized care.

Lighting design must accommodate ritual variability. Adjustable intensity, warm tones, and directional lighting allow families to create sacred zones within the room. Subtle illumination supports ceremonies such as prayer, meditation, or storytelling, without overpowering the patient's comfort or disrupting the perception of intimacy. Light becomes both functional and symbolic, signaling transitions, focus, and emotional presence.

Flooring and material choices influence ritual enactment. Nonslip surfaces, warm-touch flooring, and resilient materials accommodate barefoot movement, kneeling, or other postural practices common in many spiritual traditions. Texture, color, and acoustics subtly reinforce a sense of reverence and sacredness without overtly privileging any particular cultural system.

Spatial zoning enhances the ability to perform multiple rituals simultaneously. Micro-zones—such as the vigil zone, reflection zone, and memory zone—provide family members with discrete spaces to perform spiritual acts without interference. Movable furniture, partition screens, or floor mats facilitate temporary ritual configurations, preserving both privacy and communal participation.

The orientation of objects within the room conveys intentionality. Family members often place sacred items near the bedside, aligned with the patient's head or dominant hand. Architecturally, alcoves or dedicated surfaces can support this placement, ensuring that ritual objects are both prominent and protected. These spatial cues strengthen the emotional and symbolic resonance of the room.

Soundscapes are carefully calibrated to respect ritual activity. Adjustable ambient sound, soft background music, and acoustic isolation allow chanting, drumming, or vocal prayers to be heard clearly without causing sensory fatigue. Sound design ensures that ritual practices enrich the experience rather than create stress or distraction.

Color palettes subtly support cultural and spiritual rituals. Soft earth tones, warm neutrals, and calming blues or greens create an environment conducive to reflection and presence. Accent areas may include richer tones or symbolic colors, allowing families to enhance the emotional impact of their rituals without overwhelming the overall visual harmony.

Ritual furniture design balances flexibility and symbolic resonance. Chairs, benches, or cushions designed for kneeling, meditation, or seated reflection provide comfort while enabling participation. These elements are movable and lightweight, allowing the room's configuration to adapt dynamically to different rituals.

The integration of scent in ritual practices is carefully managed. Aromatherapy, incense, or other olfactory elements are balanced with ventilation systems to avoid overstimulation. When incorporated mindfully, scent can reinforce emotional memory, spiritual focus, and familial presence, anchoring rituals in multisensory engagement.

Rituals often unfold in temporal patterns. Dawn or dusk, specific prayer times, or transitional moments such as a final breath are integrated into family or staff routines. The room's design accommodates these temporal flows, ensuring that objects, lighting, and seating are arranged to support rituals whenever they are needed.

Staff facilitation is embedded in ritual-friendly design. Nurses and chaplains are trained to anticipate family needs, guide object placement, adjust lighting or ventilation, and provide discreet support. Architectural cues, such as clear sightlines and accessible storage, enable staff to support rituals without intruding, preserving the dignity and autonomy of family practices.

Visual hierarchy is carefully considered. Sacred objects, altars, or focal points are placed to draw attention subtly while maintaining overall spatial balance. This hierarchy allows ritual objects to communicate significance without overwhelming the functional or emotional flow of the room.

Micro-lighting for ritual spaces reinforces emotional and spiritual resonance. Small lamps, fiber-optic fixtures, or localized accent lighting allows families to focus attention on sacred acts without disrupting ambient comfort. These features support intentionality, symbolism, and presence within daily care routines.

Ritual-friendly rooms accommodate multiple traditions simultaneously. By providing neutral, adaptable zones and storage, hospice spaces can host overlapping practices, such as simultaneous meditation and prayer. Flexibility ensures inclusivity, signaling respect for all belief systems without privileging any single tradition.

Architecture responds to ritual needs not by dictating behavior but by facilitating meaningful action. Thoughtful placement of furniture, lighting, and objects creates a framework in which cultural and spiritual rituals can flourish organically, providing families and patients with space, comfort, and dignity.

Ultimately, designing for cultural and spiritual rituals ensures that the hospice environment is more than a clinical space. It becomes a vessel for relational, emotional, and symbolic expression, allowing families and staff to honor life, memory, and transition. These rituals, supported by architecture, light, objects, and sound, create an environment in which presence, love, and cultural continuity coexist seamlessly.

The moment of death in a hospice setting is both intensely intimate and profoundly ritualized. Staff, families, and the environment converge to mark the transition with gestures that are simultaneously practical, emotional, and symbolic. Each act, whether small or grand, contributes to a coherent narrative of presence, respect, and closure.

The final breath ritual is the most pivotal. As the patient exhales their last conscious breath, families and staff often align their attention to that singular moment. Hands are held, fingers intertwined, and the room's pace slows. Lighting is dimmed, either through manual adjustment or automated systems, creating a visual cue that the room has entered sacred time. Silence pervades, broken only by the subtle rhythm of breathing and the soft sounds of the room, allowing the transition to unfold without interruption.

Dimmed lighting functions as both practical and symbolic reinforcement. By lowering illumination gradually in the moments preceding and following death, staff signal the passage from active life to memory. This controlled adjustment of light mirrors natural circadian rhythms and supports the emotional framing of the event, preparing both family and staff for the transition.

The lamp ritual is one of the most visually emblematic gestures in hospice care. After the patient has passed, a bedside lamp is turned off deliberately. This act is neither hurried nor incidental; it is performed with reverence, marking the completion of the vigil and signaling a temporal closure to those who have shared the intimate space. The lamp's extinguishing is a symbolic gesture acknowledging the patient's presence, life, and the shift from care to remembrance.

Opening windows is incorporated in some cultural and spiritual traditions as a means of releasing the spirit. The gentle flow of air is interpreted as a bridge between the physical and spiritual world, facilitating the patient's departure. This ritual is subtle yet profoundly meaningful for families who understand the symbolism, providing a sensory affirmation of transition that resonates with belief and comfort.

The body-care ritual is both practical and ceremonial. Nurses and aides wash the body gently, smooth clothing or blankets, and cover the patient with a dignity blanket. Each movement is performed with attentiveness to touch, texture, and alignment, ensuring that the physical presentation of the body honors the individual's identity and preserves the emotional integrity of the moment.

Hand placement and touch during body care are crucial. Softly supporting the head, adjusting the hands, or gently folding arms over the chest conveys care, respect, and continuity. These gestures are deliberate, embodying a silent language of attention that communicates the value of the life just passed.

Arrangement of the room for the final moments is intentional. Chairs are positioned to allow family presence, objects of significance remain accessible, and lighting is balanced to support the emotional and symbolic weight of the transition. These spatial adjustments reinforce relational and environmental coherence.

The transition ritual often includes coordinated staff movement. Minimal verbal communication ensures that the room remains quiet, allowing families to process the moment without distraction. Staff bodies move with choreographed precision, handling equipment, linens, and objects in ways that maintain both dignity and emotional containment.

In certain traditions, ritual objects accompany the patient through the moment of death. Family-provided items, such as prayer beads, blankets, or symbolic stones, may remain in contact with the patient. Their presence serves as a tactile and visual affirmation of memory, love, and cultural or spiritual continuity.

The room's auditory environment is carefully modulated. Staff intentionally reduce extraneous noise, maintain soft floorings, and allow any music, chants, or whispered prayers to be heard clearly. Sound becomes a secondary layer of ritual, reinforcing emotional focus and presence.

Ritualized gestures continue even after the final breath. Straightening blankets, smoothing hair, and arranging pillows are acts that honor both the deceased and those who remain. Each motion is performed as a conscious repetition of care, transforming functional acts into symbolic acts of closure.

Lighting cues are often synchronized with these gestures. Small accent lights may remain dimmed, creating "glow pockets" that highlight ritualized spaces such as bedside tables or memory surfaces. These visual markers subtly frame the ceremonial acts, guiding attention and reinforcing the sacred nature of the moment.

The handover ritual signals the transition from private to communal acknowledgment. Staff escort the body through hallways quietly, often with a minimal team, ensuring that movement is calm, reverent, and synchronized. This ritual communicates respect not only to the patient but also to colleagues and the broader hospice community.

Spatial and temporal choreography is critical during the handover. Hallways are cleared, doors are closed softly, and staff footsteps are controlled to minimize disruption. Each movement emphasizes intentionality, demonstrating that every part of the patient's passage is attended to with purpose and dignity.

Families are often incorporated into the handover ritual. They may accompany the body briefly or participate in a silent gesture of farewell. This inclusion provides relational continuity and allows family members to witness the final phase of transition, enhancing emotional and psychological processing.

Ritualized objects may travel with the patient during the handover. Blankets, spiritual items, or personal mementos are carefully carried, ensuring that the patient's identity, values, and relational connections are honored through the spatial journey.

Staff reflections immediately following the transition are part of the broader ritual continuum. Brief debriefings, silent acknowledgments, or shared gestures of support among colleagues reinforce professional identity and emotional resilience. These acts create a secondary ritual layer that sustains the caregiving community.

The culmination of the transition ritual merges practical, emotional, and symbolic dimensions. Each element—lighting, touch, object placement, movement, and silence—coalesces into a coherent experience that validates the significance of the patient's life and the relational depth of the final moments.

Through repeated enactment of transition rituals, hospice staff cultivate a rhythm of care that transcends individual patients. These practices internalize values of dignity, presence, and reverence, shaping the culture of care and the emotional architecture of the space.

Ultimately, the transition ritual affirms that death in hospice is not a clinical endpoint but, rather, a profoundly relational and symbolic moment. Through carefully choreographed gestures, environmental adjustments, and relational attention, the hospice room becomes a vessel for presence, love, and memory—ensuring that the passage of life is acknowledged with depth, care, and enduring significance.

5
The Room as Archive

Hospice rooms function as repositories of human experience, holding both visible objects and invisible traces of care. The concept of "spatial memory" refers to the subtle accumulation of emotional residue left by repeated acts of presence, attention, and compassion. Each brush of a hand, adjustment of a blanket, or dimming of a lamp contributes to the room's history, embedding a narrative that both staff and families sense intuitively.[1] Over time, these imprints form a palpable atmosphere that communicates comfort, dignity, or, conversely, tension, creating a space that seems alive with the echoes of human relationships.

Spatial memory is distinct from haunted space. Haunted spaces often evoke unease or anxiety, stemming from neglect, inconsistent care, or disorganized environments. In contrast, hallowed spaces arise from repeated, intentional acts of attention. The calm, ritualized practices of staff—whether smoothing a pillow, adjusting lighting, or placing a familiar object on a table—infuse the environment with a sense of order, respect, and relational continuity. These practices transform the room into a sanctuary where presence and care are palpable even to those who enter for the first time.

Staff intuition plays a central role in perceiving spatial memory. Experienced nurses and aides often describe "entering a room and feeling its weight," an awareness cultivated through years of observing interactions, gestures, and emotional energy. This sensitivity allows caregivers to recognize rooms that carry a positive emotional imprint versus those that feel tense or heavy. Their responses—softening tone, adjusting the environment, or gently repositioning objects—further reinforce the positive affect embedded within the space.

Material surfaces contribute significantly to memory formation. Wood, linen, wool, and matte finishes are tactile and visually warm, signaling permanence and human scale. As these materials age, they acquire patina—slight wear patterns, softened edges, fingerprints—that serve as a visual record of repeated human presence. These subtle traces do not merely mark time; they encode the memory of care, attention, and ritualized gestures.[2]

The repetition of daily rituals amplifies spatial memory. Each act of caregiving, no matter how small—the brushing of hair, the adjustment of a blanket, or the careful placement of a cup—adds layers of meaning. Over days and weeks, these actions accumulate into a rhythm, creating an environment that feels coherent, predictable, and emotionally supportive. Families learn to anticipate these rhythms, which reinforces their sense of participation and trust in the care environment.[3]

Furniture placement reinforces memory and ritual. Chairs positioned near windows for reflection, tables for photographs or personal artifacts, and alcoves for spiritual items create distinct zones within the room. These micro-zones allow both staff and families to navigate the space intentionally, reinforcing the continuity of care and the symbolic weight of objects. Each arrangement contributes to the narrative of presence embedded in the environment.

Staff movement patterns also inscribe memory into the room. The choreography of walking to adjust lighting, check vitals, or perform bedside rituals creates a rhythm that is absorbed by the space. Over time, these repeated patterns of human movement form a "behavioral imprint," subtly cueing emotional responses and guiding family interaction. These kinetic traces complement the tactile and visual memory stored in objects and surfaces.

Family members sense this accumulated memory as well. Returning families often describe feeling "welcomed" or "comforted" upon entering a previously inhabited room, noticing familiar objects, familiar furniture arrangements, or the subtle warmth of lighting cues. This continuity reinforces a sense of relational stability, signaling that the patient's presence has been honored and that their memory remains tangible within the space.

Objects themselves serve as anchors for memory. Everyday items, such as a favorite mug, journal, or piece of jewelry, carry stories that resonate with both family and staff. The careful placement of these items transforms them from mere possessions into symbols of identity, continuity, and relational connection. Their presence strengthens the sense of the room as a lived archive rather than a sterile, functional space.

Lighting plays a central role in encoding emotional memory. Warm, diffused lighting layered throughout the room—ambient, task, and accent—creates a temporal rhythm that aligns with care practices.[4] This subtle modulation communicates attentiveness and intention, signaling to families that their loved one is being cared for with both functional competence and emotional sensitivity.

Acoustic design also shapes how memory is perceived. Rooms that minimize reverberation, absorb footsteps, and manage ambient noise allow attention to focus on human interaction and ritual.[5] The ability to hear a whispered story, a prayer, or the soft guidance of staff contributes to the room's emotional imprint, amplifying the resonance of gestures, words, and presence.

Cultural and spiritual rituals further enrich spatial memory. Practices such as chanting, meditation, prayer, or song performed repeatedly within the room embed sensory and symbolic meaning. These ritual acts leave layers of memory that extend beyond the immediate experience, helping staff and families remember and honor the patient's life long after death.[6]

Temporal markers enhance the perception of continuity. Observing natural light changes through windows, aligning caregiving with routine schedules, and timing rituals to coincide with significant moments establish patterns that reinforce emotional stability. These markers help families situate themselves within the flow of care, allowing the room itself to function as a narrative landscape of memory and presence.

Tactile qualities of the environment are also critical. Soft textiles, warm-touch flooring, and carefully selected bedding invite interaction and physical closeness. Touching a blanket, leaning against a familiar chair, or resting hands on a smooth wooden surface triggers memory and emotional grounding, reinforcing the relational context of care.

Even seemingly minor gestures contribute to the room's narrative. Straightening a blanket, adjusting a pillow, and smoothing curtains are small actions that, repeated over time, communicate consistency, attentiveness, and emotional presence. These acts ensure that the room retains a coherent emotional signature, reassuring families and signaling continuity to staff.

Family participation in shaping spatial memory is profound. By arranging photographs, letters, or symbolic items, families embed personal narratives alongside the professional care rituals. This collaborative process transforms the room into a multilayered archive that reflects both relational love and caregiving intention, creating a space that is both individualized and universally supportive.

Transitions of life and death leave unique traces in spatial memory. Rooms in which multiple patients have been cared for acquire a layered history, visible in patina, object placement, and ritualized arrangements. Staff recognize these traces and use them to inform subsequent interactions, ensuring that attention to emotional resonance is continuous.

Architectural design amplifies these effects. Ceiling height, sightlines, and window placement influence perception, orientation, and comfort. Clear spatial coherence allows rituals, objects, and human interactions to integrate seamlessly, reinforcing the positive imprint of repeated acts of presence and care.

Staff reflection and documentation further perpetuate memory. Debriefings, mentoring, and team observations codify experiential knowledge, ensuring that the emotional and relational significance of a space is recognized and preserved across shifts and caregiving teams. These practices maintain the room as an archive of care, learning, and human connection.

Ultimately, emotional residue transforms a hospice room into a living archive of life, care, and memory. Material choices, spatial coherence, ritual repetition, family engagement, and attentive presence converge to create an environment in which the absence of a patient is met with continuity, and presence resonates long after the moment of death. The room holds stories, honors identity, and becomes a vessel for the enduring human connections that define hospice care.[7]

Hospice rooms are more than physical structures; they are vessels that accumulate emotional, sensory, and relational memory over time. Each patient, each family, and each staff member contributes to a continuum of presence that lingers long after their departure. The room becomes a repository not only of objects but also of intangible traces—emotional footprints, whispered prayers, and subtle gestures of care—that collectively create an invisible community.

Families often sense the history of a room without consciously knowing why. A parent sitting beside a hospice bed may feel an unspoken comfort, a sense of continuity that comes not from the individual experience alone but from the accumulated presence of past occupants. These perceptions are subtle, rooted in an intuitive recognition that the space has been cared for, respected, and held by many before them.

Scent is a powerful vehicle for memory. Lavender spray, warm washcloths, freshly laundered linens, and the aroma of tea evoke presence and calm, anchoring families in the rhythm of care. These olfactory cues become part of the room's invisible narrative, signaling to new occupants that compassion and attentiveness are embedded in the environment. Such sensory memory operates alongside visual and tactile cues, reinforcing the emotional imprint of the space.

Sound memory also accumulates. Soft footsteps across carpeting, chairs shifting gently, whispered prayers, and the quiet tones of staff conversation layer into the auditory fabric of the room. Families entering the space can perceive this subtle resonance, often describing it as a "weight of care" or a "soft hum of attention," a phenomenon that helps them navigate grief and presence with reassurance.

The choreography of staff movement is an integral contributor to the room's invisible community. Each repeated gesture—adjusting lighting, smoothing blankets, or placing a cup of water—leaves an imprint, a silent notation that is absorbed by the room's occupants. Over time, these gestures become part of the room's narrative, an enduring record of attentiveness and care that informs subsequent interactions.

Objects, too, retain echoes of the past. A well-worn blanket, a favorite mug, or a memory surface carrying family photos absorbs more than tactile weight; it carries relational history. Staff recognize that placement and care of these objects communicate respect for both the patient and the broader lineage of care that the room holds. The room thus mediates connection across time, bridging past and present occupants.

Families often participate in these invisible rituals, sometimes unconsciously. Placing a photograph on a shelf, holding a hand in silence, or repositioning a blanket in a familiar pattern aligns with a rhythm established by previous occupants. Through these acts, the room becomes a communal space of emotional continuity, a living archive in which human presence transcends individual experiences.

Light, as a medium, contributes to the room's accumulated presence. Diffused bedside illumination, the soft glow of an overhead lamp, or indirect natural light entering through a window carries residual memory of care routines and vigil practices. Families may sense that these lighting patterns are intentional, reinforcing the impression that the room has been thoughtfully prepared for meaningful engagement.

Spatial arrangement supports the invisible community. Chairs, alcoves, and zones for ritualized activities are rarely neutral; their placement reflects both functional necessity and relational memory. Returning families intuitively use these spaces in ways established by previous occupants, aligning their actions with an inherited choreography that supports emotional presence and engagement.

The invisible community also includes subtle psychological cues. The room's calm energy, the quiet order of objects, and the deliberate pacing of staff movement communicate reassurance and stability. Families unconsciously read these cues, which guide their emotional responses, facilitate grieving, and reinforce the sense that they are part of a lineage of care and attention.

Sound layering enhances emotional memory. Even when the room is empty, residual acoustic impressions—soft echoes of previous conversations, the gentle tapping of a nurse's shoes on the floor, the rhythm of ventilated airflow—create an ambient familiarity. These auditory cues enrich the room's narrative, offering an emotional guide for both staff and family during critical moments of presence.

The invisible community is also shaped by temporal repetition. Observing natural light transitions, the cadence of care routines, and predictable ritual timing reinforces the memory of previous interactions. Families experience continuity because the room carries patterns established by repeated human action, making even first-time visits feel coherent and welcoming.

Touch is another medium for spatial memory. Tactile engagement with blankets, linens, furniture, and personal objects reinforces emotional connection. Families and staff perceive these touch-mediated memories as comforting, conveying a sense of shared care across time. Each gesture adds a layer to the room's ongoing narrative, contributing to the invisible archive of presence.

Cultural and spiritual practices extend the invisible community's reach. Prayer, song, chanting, and other ceremonial acts leave traces that can be sensed even by subsequent occupants who may not share the same tradition. The room thus mediates cross-cultural memory, supporting diverse families and care teams while maintaining continuity of relational care.

The rhythm of caregiving further embeds memory. Subtle patterns in staff routines—approaching the bedside, adjusting lighting, offering hydration, and speaking softly—create a temporal framework that families absorb. These rhythms link past and present experiences, allowing new occupants to navigate the room emotionally as part of a continuing legacy.

The room's materiality reinforces invisible memory. Soft textiles, matte finishes, natural wood, and muted surfaces serve as tactile repositories of interaction. They absorb gestures, weights, and contact patterns, providing sensory evidence of previous presence that informs the perceptions and actions of current occupants.

Even after a patient has passed, the invisible community persists. The careful arrangement of personal items, lingering scents, and maintained furniture positions serve as transitional memory anchors for families, signaling that presence continues beyond physical absence. Staff intentionally preserve these cues to support grief processing and relational continuity.

Staff reflection and team memory are integral to the room's invisible community. Debriefings and mentoring ensure that the subtleties of emotional and spatial presence are communicated across shifts. This professional memory preserves relational knowledge, ensuring that new teams understand the room's history and act with consistent care and sensitivity.

The invisible community ultimately transforms the hospice room into a relational archive. Each sensory cue—scent, touch, sound, light, and object placement—interweaves with human action to create a persistent memory landscape. Families and staff experience the room as simultaneously private and communal, personal and shared, reflecting the cumulative care of countless lives.

This phenomenon demonstrates that hospice spaces function not merely as neutral containers but as active participants in caregiving. By holding echoes of past interactions, the room mediates emotional connection, supports ritualized practice, and fosters relational continuity across time. In doing so, it ensures that the essence of presence endures, sustaining memory, care, and dignity in every visit.

Hospice rooms must navigate the delicate balance between personal memory and spatial clarity. Designing for memory without clutter requires creating spaces that can hold the emotional weight of a life while remaining functionally navigable for staff and comfortable for families. A room that is overcrowded with personal items, photographs, and memorabilia can overwhelm the senses, increasing stress for both the dying patient and their loved ones. Conversely, a room with no personal anchors can feel sterile, alienating, and emotionally barren

Memory-friendly architecture begins with a sense of warmth and openness. Materials such as natural wood, soft textiles, and matte finishes signal comfort and human scale, and clear sightlines and logical spatial arrangements maintain clarity. Even when families bring multiple objects, the architecture provides "breathing space," allowing each item to be meaningful without creating visual chaos.

Surface design is central to balancing memory and order. Bedside tables, shelves, and alcoves are deliberately scaled to accommodate personal items such as photos, letters, or small mementos while discouraging overcrowding. Surfaces that invite touch and interaction—such as smooth wood, linen mats, and soft trays—encourage family engagement and tactile connection without compromising functional space.

Boundaries for personalization are essential. Frames, shallow shelves, or designated display areas provide implicit limits, ensuring that emotional expression does not overwhelm the room. These boundaries are not restrictive; rather, they guide families to curate meaningful items intentionally, reinforcing the significance of each object and maintaining a sense of calm and coherence.

Modular storage solutions allow for both flexibility and discretion. Drawers, cabinets, and concealed compartments provide space for clinical tools, personal effects, or temporary items while keeping the room visually uncluttered. Staff can maintain functionality without encroaching on the emotional resonance of the space, ensuring that both care and memory coexist harmoniously.

Flexible wall space offers an adaptable canvas for temporary personalization. Families may hang photographs, cards, or children's drawings on magnetic boards, clips, or light rails. These items become temporal extensions of memory, allowing families to express love and connection while ensuring that the room can revert to a neutral state after the patient passes.

The distinction between curated memory and emotional overload is subtle but profound. Curated memory focuses attention on a few deeply meaningful items, enhancing reflection, connection, and comfort. Emotional overload, by contrast, saturates the senses with too many objects, colors, or stimuli, potentially inducing anxiety or distraction. Thoughtful architectural and design choices prevent this, maintaining an environment conducive to attentional focus and presence.

Lighting strategies also reinforce memory without clutter. Accent lighting can illuminate specific objects or surfaces, drawing attention to meaningful items without creating visual noise. Adjustable bedside lamps and soft indirect lighting provide intimacy, allowing families to focus on memory-rich objects while preserving the room's broader calm.

Textural layering contributes to emotional resonance. A well-chosen blanket, pillow, or rug can anchor memory, providing tactile reassurance. Such textiles should be chosen for warmth and comfort, not sheer abundance, ensuring that the space remains navigable and calming while offering sensory cues that reinforce attachment and presence.

Furniture placement supports both functional flow and memory display. Chairs, tables, and alcoves are arranged to encourage engagement with objects without impeding movement for staff or visitors. For example, a chair near a window might hold a family's memory tray, while a side table adjacent to the bed accommodates essential clinical tools discretely, maintaining a balance between presence and care.

The emotional impact of surface hierarchy is significant. Elevated surfaces or designated display areas imply importance, guiding family focus and highlighting key items. Lower surfaces for transient or everyday objects allow practical use while subtly reinforcing the primacy of memorialized items. This hierarchy prevents cognitive overload, helping families feel grounded rather than overwhelmed.

Integration of modular and temporary elements allows the room to evolve with the patient's needs. Lightweight shelves, clipboards, or magnetic panels can be added or removed as the family brings new items. This adaptability fosters a dynamic sense of participation, ensuring that the room can respond to changing emotional and ritual needs without creating permanent clutter.

Storage that conceals clinical equipment contributes to emotional clarity. Oxygen tubing, monitors, and medication kits can be integrated into cabinetry or under-bed compartments, ensuring that the room communicates warmth and care rather than clinical sterility. Families perceive the room as safe, intimate, and inviting rather than mechanical or alien.

Spatial zones help families and staff navigate emotional and functional demands. Memory zones, clinical zones, and reflection zones can coexist without interference. A small table near the bed may hold personal objects for tactile engagement, while adjacent areas provide access for staff interventions. These zones preserve dignity, minimize disruption, and maintain the integrity of both memory and care.

The placement of objects for children or extended family members deserves special attention. Lightweight, safe surfaces for artwork, cards, or small toys allow younger visitors to participate in the ritual of presence without creating clutter or compromising safety. This inclusion enhances the sense of shared community and preserves emotional coherence across generations.

Visual simplicity enhances the impact of memory-rich objects. By limiting background distractions and emphasizing a small number of meaningful items, designers ensure that each object is noticed and emotionally resonant. This focus allows families to engage deeply with their memories and rituals, reinforcing comfort and connection.

Text and imagery can be temporary and modular. Magnetic photo boards, clip displays, or replaceable frames allow families to rotate meaningful content without altering permanent room fixtures. This flexibility ensures that memory expression remains adaptive, personal, and manageable within the room's architecture.

Even small design cues contribute to perceived order. Recessed shelves, framed display areas, and subtle visual boundaries encourage thoughtful placement of personal items. These cues guide families toward curating meaningful memory while maintaining the functional integrity of the room.

Staff guidance complements architectural design. Educating families on the intended use of display areas, storage, and modular elements reinforces the balance between emotional expression and environmental clarity. This guidance ensures that memory-rich personalization remains intentional rather than accidental or overwhelming.

Ultimately, designing for memory without clutter is an exercise in emotional and spatial intelligence. Architecture, material choice, and spatial layout mediate the room's capacity to hold human stories, providing a canvas that supports family engagement, ritual, and reflection without overwhelming or distracting. Through thoughtful balance, the hospice room becomes both archive and sanctuary, capable of honoring life, memory, and presence in a coherent, calming environment.

Time in hospice spaces is a fluid, almost malleable presence. Unlike in clinical or institutional settings in which schedules and clocks dominate, the perception of time in end-of-life spaces stretches, compresses, and even dissolves depending on the emotional intensity of the moment, the patient's condition, and the family's engagement. A carefully designed hospice room recognizes this elasticity and uses architecture, materials, and spatial rhythm to guide, calm, and support those within it. In this sense, time itself becomes an architectural material, shaping experience in profound and nuanced ways.

Families often describe vigil periods as a paradoxical stretch of moments, where minutes expand into hours and hours into what feels like minutes. Architects and designers respond to this by creating subtle spatial cues that reinforce temporal orientation without imposing strict schedules. These cues include light transitions, sightlines, and material choices that gently signal the passage of the day while allowing the experience to remain human-centered and emotionally sensitive.

Natural light is among the most powerful markers of temporal continuity. Carefully placed windows, skylights, and clerestory openings provide soft, indirect light that tracks the sun's movement across the sky. Sunrise gently illuminates the room's contours, afternoon light warms the surfaces, and sunset casts long shadows that create a sense of transition. These temporal markers are absorbed subconsciously, providing reassurance and a sense of rhythm to families and patients alike.

Artificial light complements these natural cues, offering precision and control over temporal perception. Tunable lamps, indirect ceiling lighting, and accent lights allow staff to subtly adjust intensity and color, reinforcing phases of the day or signaling transitions such as rest, reflection, or vigil periods. Families may not consciously note these adjustments, but the cumulative effect contributes to a structured sense of time that supports emotional processing.

Slow architecture is a cornerstone of temporal design. The deliberate scaling of space, the gentle proportioning of ceilings, and the strategic arrangement of furniture all contribute to a deceleration of the room's pace. By designing for quiet movement and contemplative engagement, the room allows moments to linger, supporting mindfulness and encouraging the family to inhabit time rather than be rushed by it.

Materials also play a subtle but profound role in temporal perception. Textures that develop patina—soft woods, woven textiles, and matte stone surfaces—record traces of use, embedding the passage of moments in physical form. These surfaces absorb gestures and interactions, creating a layered temporal memory that reassures both staff and family that care has been continuous and present over time.

Furniture placement mediates temporal experience by directing movement and attention. Chairs near windows, reflection zones, and memory surfaces invite contemplative pause, whereas bedside seating and alcoves facilitate sustained presence during critical moments. The arrangement encourages families to slow down, observe, and engage, structuring the subjective flow of time in alignment with care rituals.

Ritual repetition is another mechanism for temporal anchoring. Staff gestures such as adjusting lighting, repositioning blankets, and offering hydration are repeated with deliberate cadence. Families quickly learn the rhythm of these gestures, absorbing the temporal flow implicitly. Each repetition builds predictability, continuity, and reassurance, transforming the perception of time from a linear measurement into an experiential phenomenon.

Sound contributes meaningfully to the perception of temporal continuity. Subtle echoes of footsteps, soft whispers, and the rhythmic hum of ventilation provide a constant auditory backdrop. Even in moments of quiet, these layered sounds create an unconscious framework, enabling families and staff to situate themselves temporally and emotionally within the room.

The subjective slowing of time intensifies during vigil hours. Families often report heightened awareness, noting each breath, each touch, and every nuanced facial expression. Architecture amplifies this by offering quiet, distraction-free zones and soft lighting that allows them to inhabit each moment fully, fostering presence and attentive care.

Conversely, temporal compression occurs when urgent interventions or unexpected events demand rapid response. Staff must maintain efficiency without disturbing the room's emotional rhythm. Clear sightlines, intuitive storage, and unobstructed circulation pathways allow essential tasks to occur seamlessly, preserving the perceived calm while meeting clinical needs.

The deliberate removal of the room's clock after a patient passes is a symbolic gesture that reinforces the timelessness of death. This act shifts focus from chronological measurement to relational and emotional presence, subtly signaling that time, as previously measured, has become irrelevant, and the focus now is on memory, ritual, and dignity.

Material finishes also influence the perception of time. Matte surfaces, muted colors, and soft textures slow visual processing, fostering a sense of calm and temporal expansion. Bright, reflective surfaces or jarring contrasts accelerate perception and create subtle stress cues, underscoring the importance of thoughtful material selection to support desired temporal experiences.

Spatial layering further mediates perception of time. Zones for reflection, vigil, and clinical care create nested temporal spaces. A chair by the window invites lingering contemplation, whereas the bedside allows attentive engagement. These nested areas provide cues about when to act, when to pause, and when to reflect, supporting both functional and emotional navigation of time.

Timed light transitions enhance circadian alignment, particularly in patients experiencing disorientation, sundowning, or terminal delirium. Gradual dimming in the evening and soft illumination in the morning cue the body and mind, reinforcing temporal continuity even in the absence of conscious awareness.

Staff movements themselves constitute a temporal rhythm. Repeated acts—such as adjusting blankets, checking vitals, and softly speaking—create an invisible choreography. Families internalize this rhythm, perceiving time as structured, gentle, and compassionate. These movements act as an emotional metronome, guiding attention and presence.

Family rituals intersect with temporal architecture to reinforce subjective time. Handholding, storytelling, journaling, prayer, and silent observation establish patterns that span minutes, hours, and days. The room, through design and layout, accommodates these temporal acts, supporting continuity of engagement and reflection.

The room's sensory and architectural design encourages families to inhabit time rather than be hurried through it. Elements such as texture, lighting, acoustics, and spatial proportion collectively create an experience in which subjective time slows, stretching moments of connection, grief, and remembrance.

Ultimately, hospice rooms designed with temporal awareness transform human experience. Time becomes an active participant in care, shaping perception, emotion, and memory. Families report feeling anchored, able to inhabit moments fully, and supported in their vigil. The space's design ensures that time is neither adversarial nor mechanical but, rather, becomes a conduit for presence, ritual, and emotional continuity.

Through this careful orchestration of spatial, sensory, and ritual elements, hospice architecture acknowledges the fluidity of time at life's end. By manipulating perception subtly and supporting families' engagement with the passing of moments, these spaces offer dignity, coherence, and sanctuary even in the face of inevitable finality.

A hospice room is more than a container of human bodies; it is a participant in the work of care, memory, and emotional continuity. Through its architecture, lighting, and carefully considered objects, the room becomes a witness to human transition, silently holding the accumulation of presence, grief, and ritual over time. Each corner, surface, and window absorbs gestures and whispers, creating a repository of the subtle, often invisible acts of devotion that define the hospice experience.

Volunteers and staff frequently serve as narrative bridges, connecting the room's history to the current occupant. Stories of past patients—anonymized to preserve privacy—help new families navigate the unfamiliar territory of impending loss. These narratives often highlight ordinary acts of courage, love, and connection, grounding the family in the continuity of human experience. The room, in this sense, functions as a participant: It holds these echoes, giving weight and resonance to each story.

Objects left temporarily after death acquire profound significance. A single flower, a favorite blanket, or a photograph can act as a storytelling anchor. Families often linger near these items, sharing memories or reflecting silently. The architecture accommodates these interactions, providing surfaces, alcoves, or niches that encourage pause, observation, and ritual without overwhelming the functional needs of the room.

Spatial design outside the room supports story-keeping as well. Quiet lounges, debrief areas, and volunteer spaces allow staff to share narratives, exchange observations, and reflect on emotional experiences without disrupting families. These areas reinforce a culture of storytelling that sustains professional resilience while honoring the room's role as a witness.

The ethical dimension of story-keeping is central. Architects and staff must balance the room's capacity to bear witness with respect for the current patient's dignity and privacy. Storytelling practices are carefully mediated: Histories are anonymized, narratives are framed to comfort rather than alarm, and objects are curated with sensitivity to emotional impact.

Memory surfaces—shelves, tables, and alcoves—become temporary archives for storytelling. Objects placed on these surfaces carry layered meaning: A family photo can prompt recollection, a handwritten card may anchor emotion, and small ritual items can convey cultural significance. The room itself is designed to highlight these items, using light, scale, and placement to underscore their importance while avoiding clutter.

The architecture communicates silently through proportion, texture, and sightlines. A window overlooking a garden can invite reflection, a soft chair near the bed signals a space for vigil, and unobstructed circulation allows gentle movement that mirrors the flow of human experience. These design choices subtly shape the narrative rhythm of the room, supporting both memory and emotional processing.

Soundscapes within the room contribute to its witness role. The hushed cadence of footsteps, the shifting of chairs, and the whispered prayers or quiet conversation all accumulate into a temporal layer that amplifies the storytelling function. Families intuitively absorb these sonic cues, interpreting the room's rhythms as part of the narrative of presence and care.

Temporal design intersects with story-keeping. The subjective stretching of moments, the elongation of vigil hours, and the gentle marking of transitions through light and ritual create conditions in which narratives can unfold naturally. Time, as felt within the room, becomes a medium through which stories are remembered, repeated, and internalized.

Staff engagement with storytelling is deliberate and ritualized. Huddles before entering a room, whispered observations during vigil hours, or reflective notes in charts serve to sustain memory continuity. These small acts ensure that stories are not lost, that the room's witness function is honored, and that each patient's presence leaves a trace beyond their physical departure.

Ethnographic studies of hospice care highlight the profound impact of storytelling on family experience. Hearing accounts of previous patients' final days can normalize fear, reduce anxiety, and model rituals of presence. The room, by accommodating these narratives through design cues and object placement, becomes an active facilitator of emotional learning.

The placement of objects can be deliberately choreographed to support narrative flow. Items that signal milestones—such as a favorite blanket, a bedside journal, or a ritual object—can cue reflection or storytelling. Families often respond intuitively, sharing anecdotes or observing quietly, creating a dynamic dialogue between presence, memory, and space.

Lighting amplifies the room's witness function. Accent lighting on objects of personal significance draws attention to their symbolic value. Soft, indirect illumination encourages reflective engagement and highlights narrative anchors without creating harsh contrasts or visual distraction.

Architectural thresholds—the first view into the room, unobstructed doorways, and visual sightlines—shape the reception of narrative and memory. A thoughtfully positioned window, a framed photograph, or a softly glowing lamp can signal the room's role as a repository of stories, inviting families to participate in its witness function.

Story-keeping extends to multigenerational memory. Children and grandchildren can contribute temporary objects—drawings, small toys, or letters—that become part of the room's archive. The architecture accommodates these contributions safely and respectfully, allowing the space to bear witness to layers of life beyond the immediate patient–family dyad.

Spatial flexibility supports narrative engagement. Modular furniture, movable shelving, and adaptable display areas allow families to curate objects in ways that reflect personal stories, cultural rituals, or spiritual beliefs. The room's design encourages this participation while maintaining functionality and clarity.

Emotional hygiene is intertwined with story-keeping. Spaces for staff reflection, debriefing, and quiet observation ensure that narrative transmission does not become burdensome or traumatic. By providing architecture that supports emotional processing, the hospice environment sustains its witness role responsibly.

Temporal markers—lighting transitions, ritual gestures, and repeated caregiving acts—reinforce narrative continuity. Families experience these as both rhythm and story, linking past, present, and anticipated moments. Architecture, objects, and staff practice converge to create a coherent narrative field.

Ultimately, hospice rooms designed as witnesses transform human experience. They carry the weight of presence, ritual, and memory, providing continuity across multiple occupants while maintaining dignity for each individual. Objects, light, sound, and spatial arrangement converge to create a living archive that participates in care, memory, and the ethical transmission of human stories.

Through this integration of design, ritual, and storytelling, the room becomes more than a site of dying. It functions as a sacred vessel, holding life's final acts, preserving emotional continuity, and offering families a space in which stories can unfold, be witnessed, and endure beyond the immediate moment.

6
A Blueprint for the Quiet Room of the Future

The foundation of a hospice room designed for peace begins with an understanding that architecture is not simply functional—it is inherently emotional. Every wall, ceiling, and floor has the capacity to influence mood, cognition, and physiological response. Soft geometry and clear sightlines are central to creating a calming environment. Rounded corners, gentle curves, and unobstructed visual axes reduce stress and minimize the potential for disorientation, especially for patients with cognitive decline or terminal delirium.[1]

Clutter-free sightlines extend beyond aesthetics; they signal safety and predictability. When family members enter a room and see the bed, window, and seating areas arranged without obstruction, they instinctively understand the spatial hierarchy and the flow of care. Emotional predictability emerges from repeated exposure to a consistent layout across multiple rooms, reinforcing comfort and reducing anxiety for both families and staff.

Material honesty is another cornerstone of peaceful design. Using natural materials such as birch, oak, wool, linen, and stone creates a tactile and visual warmth that synthetic substitutes cannot replicate. These materials age gracefully, developing patina over time, which provides subtle cues of continuity and memory. The aging of materials mirrors the life cycle, creating resonance with the human experience unfolding within the room.

Spatial planning around the bed is critical. End-of-life rituals often involve multiple participants—family members, nurses, aides, and chaplains—engaging in intimate, highly emotional acts. A spacious perimeter around the bed allows movement without obstruction, providing dignity for the patient while giving caregivers and loved ones room to perform their roles with ease. This planning also prevents feelings of crowding or confinement that can increase stress.

Cultural sensitivity is embedded into foundational architectural principles. The orientation of the bed, placement of windows, and provision of flexible wall surfaces must accommodate a variety of spiritual and cultural rituals. By incorporating this flexibility from the outset, designers honor diverse beliefs and ensure that every family can enact their traditions with dignity and comfort.[2]

Light is an integral component of peaceful architecture. Ceiling height, window placement, and the integration of indirect lighting establish both visual comfort and emotional tone. Soft, diffused light eliminates harsh shadows and glare, reducing physiological stress and creating an environment conducive to reflection and vigil.

Acoustic considerations are equally important. Sound-absorbing wall panels, soft flooring, and minimized mechanical noise prevent sensory overload. Silence becomes a carefully engineered feature, providing a canvas for human interaction rather than a vacuum, and allowing whispered conversations, prayers, and vigil rituals to resonate meaningfully within the room.

Sightlines must be choreographed to balance openness with intimacy. A patient should not be immediately visible upon entering the room; instead, the view should unfold gently, emphasizing nature, art, or light before revealing the bed. This sequencing reduces initial shock, honors dignity, and establishes a gentle entry into the sacred temporal space of end-of-life care.

The integration of memory surfaces—tables, shelves, and alcoves—must align with principles of peace. These surfaces provide space for photographs, ritual objects, or personal items while maintaining clear movement pathways and visual calm. Design attention to proportion, height, and placement ensures that these objects contribute to emotional presence without creating clutter or distraction.

Furniture selection reflects both ergonomics and psychological comfort. Chairs with gentle support, adjustable seating, and fabric that invites touch encourage family members to linger. Beds should balance clinical functionality with homelike aesthetics, avoiding cold, institutional cues that can disrupt the perception of serenity.

Circulation patterns are subtle yet crucial. Hallways, door thresholds, and intra-room pathways are designed to minimize congestion, reduce accidental contact, and support intuitive movement. Families and staff instinctively sense these pathways, reducing cognitive load and enhancing the room's calm influence.

Color palettes contribute to emotional predictability. Soft neutrals, warm earth tones, and muted accent colors reduce visual tension, enhance material warmth, and provide a consistent aesthetic language across multiple rooms. This predictability fosters trust and comfort for both new and returning families.

Storage solutions are integrated seamlessly. Clinical tools, personal items, and ritual objects must be accessible without visual disruption. Concealed cabinetry, modular shelving, and adaptive storage solutions allow for functional efficiency while maintaining the room's peaceful character.

Spatial hierarchy is deliberately considered. Reflection zones, vigil chairs, staff alcoves, and bedside access are proportioned to support varied temporal and emotional rhythms. Each zone's design communicates its purpose without signage, relying on subtle cues such as scale, orientation, and surface treatment to guide behavior.

Ventilation and air quality are designed to reduce stress and support comfort. Quiet air circulation, temperature stability, and the inclusion of natural elements—such as indoor plants or views to gardens—anchor occupants in a sensory environment conducive to presence and reflection.

Integration of flexible technology is subtle but essential. Monitoring equipment, lighting controls, and environmental adjustments are accessible yet unobtrusive, allowing staff to provide clinical care without disrupting the room's emotional tone. These invisible interventions ensure that peace is maintained even amid medical activity.

The principle of modular adaptability supports diverse rituals. Furniture, shelving, and partitions can be adjusted to accommodate spiritual practices, family preferences, or specific bedside configurations. This flexibility signals respect for autonomy, enhancing both dignity and emotional comfort.

Art and visual elements are curated to support tranquility. Landscapes, abstracts, or culturally meaningful imagery are strategically placed to encourage reflection without imposing narrative or distraction. Visual focus points create resting spaces for the eyes and mind, reinforcing calm and temporal continuity.

Finally, the architecture fosters a sense of sanctuary. Every design choice—from material selection and light placement to circulation and spatial hierarchy—works together to create a space that communicates safety, dignity, and presence. The quiet room becomes more than a functional environment; it becomes a vessel for emotional, spiritual, and human continuity, embodying the principles of peaceful architecture that sustain patients, families, and staff through the profound intensity of end-of-life care.

Hospice rooms are unique spaces in which the needs of patients, families, and staff intersect, often simultaneously and with intensity. Designing such a space requires recognizing that each group brings distinct physical, emotional, and psychological demands, and that the architecture itself can mediate, harmonize, and sometimes buffer these competing requirements. A room that succeeds in balancing these needs becomes more than a functional environment: It becomes a vessel for presence, memory, ritual, and care, holding the weight of human experience in ways that are both subtle and profound.

At the center of design considerations are patient needs. Patients at the end of life face vulnerability, fear, and sensory overload. A thoughtfully designed room can reduce these stressors through clarity, predictability, and sensory comfort. Soft geometric forms, unobstructed sightlines, and an organized layout communicate stability and safety, reducing cognitive and emotional strain. Orientation cues, such as window placement or gentle light gradients, anchor the patient in time and space, offering a subtle counterbalance to the disorienting aspects of illness or delirium.

Sensory comfort encompasses multiple modalities. Patients may be hypersensitive to light, sound, or touch. Materials such as warm wood, soft textiles, and matte surfaces create a tactile environment that reassures and soothes, while acoustic considerations—sound-absorbing panels, quiet flooring, and mechanical noise reduction—allow the patient to experience a quiet, meditative atmosphere. Each element is deliberately chosen to reduce distress, create predictability, and encourage relaxation, even in the final hours.

Spatial planning around the bed must account for both human presence and procedural needs. End-of-life rituals, caregiving activities, and medical interventions require ample space for movement without crowding or obstruction. Beds positioned with generous clearance allow family members to gather for vigil, staff to perform care unobtrusively, and patients to experience dignity and agency within the constraints of their condition. This spatial generosity signals respect, comfort, and emotional containment simultaneously.

Families also require carefully considered space. They often spend long hours at the bedside, sometimes overnight, and need areas to sit, rest, and engage in rituals or reflection. Chairs, small sofas, and fold-out sleeping solutions must be thoughtfully placed to maintain visibility of the patient while allowing family members private space for conversation, journaling, or quiet contemplation. The room must support their physical endurance as well as their emotional and spiritual presence.

Grieving families require zones that feel safe for both engagement and withdrawal. Some may wish to be fully present at the bedside; others may need a quiet corner to process emotions, speak with staff, or rest briefly. By providing spatial differentiation—vigil zones, reflection corners, and flexible seating arrangements—the architecture accommodates these varying needs without diminishing the family's ability to connect with the patient.

Staff needs intersect with both patient and family requirements, but their demands are primarily functional. Clear circulation paths, ergonomic furniture, and immediate access to medical supplies support efficiency and safety. Staff must be able to provide urgent care, administer medication, or respond to changes in condition without disrupting the emotional and ritual flow of the room. When these pathways are carefully designed, the room supports care while maintaining dignity and emotional calm for all occupants.

Dual-purpose walls are an effective strategy for balancing these overlapping requirements. These walls conceal clinical tools, storage, and utilities while simultaneously offering soft visual cues, such as niches, textures, or accent lighting, that reinforce calm and emotional resonance. By integrating functional and emotional elements within the same architectural feature, designers can prevent visual clutter and maintain continuity of experience across different users of the space.

Lighting strategies in a multi-sided space must accommodate simultaneous needs. Adjustable ambient, task, and accent lighting ensures that staff can perform clinical duties, families can read or reflect, and patients experience gentle illumination that promotes rest and comfort. Layered lighting allows the room to adapt dynamically to varying moments, signaling transition from caregiving to vigil or facilitating intimate family interactions without imposing harsh illumination.

Acoustic management is equally crucial. Staff conversations, family whispers, mechanical noises, and the subtle sounds of caregiving accumulate in a small room. Sound-absorbing materials, quiet floors, and deliberate separation of activity zones prevent sensory conflict, allowing each participant to engage without feeling overwhelmed. The architecture shapes an auditory environment that supports presence, memory, and calm.

Spatial zoning supports multiple layers of activity. The patient zone, reflection zone, and staff alcove are proportioned according to anticipated use, creating intuitive guidance without the need for signage. Families naturally understand where to sit or stand, staff can move efficiently, and patients retain both dignity and autonomy. These zones intersect yet do not conflict, allowing a harmonious coexistence that preserves peace and function simultaneously.

Furniture selection embodies the needs of all groups. Chairs, beds, and work surfaces are chosen for ergonomics, durability, and aesthetic warmth. Seating encourages family members to linger; beds provide comfort and clinical access; and staff surfaces support safe, efficient workflows. Each piece contributes to the room's overall balance of function, comfort, and emotional resonance, ensuring that design decisions reflect human experience rather than purely technical requirements.

Materiality communicates subtle signals across all participants. Warm, natural surfaces reassure patients and families, while easy-to-clean finishes maintain hygiene for staff. The juxtaposition of tactile warmth and clinical efficiency embodies the room's multi-sided character, balancing the emotional and functional dimensions without compromise.

Flexibility underpins the accommodation of cultural and spiritual practices. Movable partitions, modular furniture, and adaptable memory surfaces allow families to configure the space according to personal rituals, while staff can maintain operational efficiency. The architecture itself acts as a mediator, enabling variability without sacrificing visual order or calm, fostering an environment that honors diverse traditions and practices.

Storage solutions must be both functional and discreet. Concealed cabinetry hides medical supplies and equipment, ensuring they remain accessible to staff yet invisible to families and patients. Open surfaces provide temporary space for personal items, ritual objects, or storytelling anchors, supporting both presence and emotional continuity. This careful balance reduces clutter while preserving the room's narrative and ritual potential.

Environmental control is critical for all occupants. Patients may have heightened sensitivity to temperature or airflow, families require comfort during extended stays, and staff need a stable environment for clinical work. Zoning heating, ventilation, and air-conditioning systems, quiet air circulation, and subtle climate controls ensure that all participants experience comfort without distraction or conflict.

Sightline management maintains dignity, privacy, and intuitive guidance. Families can observe the patient without feeling intrusive, staff can monitor care discreetly, and patients retain a sense of autonomy and control. Strategic furniture placement, partitioning, and room orientation support these overlapping visual needs, reducing stress and friction.

Temporal design aligns with the rhythms of multiple users. Lighting transitions, material cues, and designated ritual zones provide structure for vigil hours, caregiving sequences, and family interactions. By framing these temporal flows architecturally, the room supports coherence and emotional continuity without imposing rigidity.

Ultimately, the multi-sided hospice room embodies a convergence of functional, emotional, and cultural needs into a coherent, harmonious environment. Thoughtful architecture, dual-purpose solutions, and intuitive spatial cues transform potential friction into a fluid, empathetic coexistence. The room communicates permission, containment, and flexibility, allowing patients, families, and staff to coexist peacefully during one of life's most intense transitions.

By mediating the needs of all participants, the room becomes a silent participant in care, a witness to ritual, and a vessel for presence. Its architecture supports dignity, emotional expression, and functional efficiency simultaneously, demonstrating how design can actively shape the experience of the end of life, not merely accommodate it.

Hospice rooms must anticipate unpredictability. Each patient's end-of-life journey is unique, influenced by medical trajectory, emotional state, family composition, and cultural or spiritual practices. Flexibility is therefore a foundational principle of design, allowing the room to accommodate a wide spectrum of rituals, gathering sizes, and sensory needs without compromising comfort or dignity.

Movable furniture is an essential element in achieving this adaptability. Chairs, tables, and even small beds can be designed for easy reconfiguration, allowing the space to expand or contract according to the number of family members present or the type of ritual being performed. This mobility enables cultural practices such as prayer circles, dance, or storytelling to unfold organically within the room, preserving both the sanctity of the ritual and the functionality of the care environment.

Spatial openness is particularly important when families arrive in groups. Extended families, friends, or faith leaders may all wish to participate in vigil or final rites. By providing flexible furniture and modular seating, the room can accommodate multiple participants without overcrowding, maintaining a sense of calm while honoring diverse traditions. Families instinctively understand that the space can adapt to their presence, reinforcing a feeling of agency and comfort during a highly emotional time.

Technology can be integrated subtly to support these adaptable needs. Soundscapes, for example, allow families to introduce culturally or spiritually meaningful music without disturbing the patient or clinical workflow. Dimming automation can transition the room from caregiving brightness to vigil-level intimacy, signaling the shift from daily care to reflective presence. Silent call systems permit staff to respond quickly to patient needs while minimizing disruption, preserving the room's peaceful atmosphere.

Multigenerational considerations are often overlooked, yet they are critical in hospice spaces. Children may accompany parents or grandparents, and the room must accommodate their physical and emotional needs. Low seating, soft floor mats, or small activity areas allow children to sit, draw, or observe vigil without interfering with adult participation. Providing for younger family members reduces stress on parents and allows them to engage fully in caregiving and ritual practices.

Flexibility also serves trauma-informed design. In cases of sudden death, unexpected medical crises, or complicated grief, staff must be able to adjust the environment to meet urgent needs without disturbing the family unnecessarily. Movable partitions, quiet zones, and modular storage allow for rapid adaptation, creating a sense of control and containment even amid emotional upheaval.

Material selection intersects with flexibility. Durable, lightweight furniture and modular finishes allow the room to be rearranged frequently without wear or damage. Surfaces that are both tactile and resilient ensure that objects can be moved, placed, or rearranged in service of ritual without losing warmth or visual cohesion. Families and staff alike respond positively to these subtle cues of adaptability.

Lighting systems must be equally flexible. Tunable, layered illumination enables multiple activities to occur simultaneously. Families can engage in conversation, reflection, or prayer while staff perform care tasks unnoticed. Adjustable bedside lamps, ambient ceiling lighting, and accent lights for memory surfaces or ritual objects create a multilayered environment in which each user can control the visual field to suit their emotional and functional needs.

Acoustic flexibility is equally critical. Families may wish to chant, pray, or speak softly, while staff may need to communicate medical updates or perform procedures. Sound-absorbing surfaces, zoned acoustics, and quiet mechanical systems allow these overlapping soundscapes to coexist without conflict, preserving the emotional tone of the room.

Storage and concealment must be adaptable. Clinical tools, ritual items, and family mementos can coexist within the room if storage is modular and discreet. Dual-purpose cabinetry or hidden niches allow objects to be accessed or stowed depending on the current activity, maintaining both functional readiness and visual serenity.

The ability to transform the room supports cultural and spiritual diversity. Some faiths require directional alignment, movement during prayer, or placement of ritual objects. Flexible spatial design allows families to configure the room according to these practices without needing structural modifications, signaling respect for autonomy and belief.

Staff benefit directly from a flexible environment. Reduced physical barriers, clear sightlines, and adaptive furniture minimize strain during caregiving, while also reducing the emotional stress of managing large families or complex rituals. A room that can accommodate multiple scenarios prevents friction and allows staff to focus on human-centered care rather than logistical problem-solving.

Flexibility also addresses temporal variability. A room may be used for several days of care, during which activity levels fluctuate dramatically. The same space that serves as a clinical setting during the day can become a vigil area in the evening, and a reflection or memory space overnight. Each shift in purpose is facilitated by movable furniture, adjustable lighting, and modular surfaces, making transitions seamless for all occupants.

Memory surfaces—tables, shelves, and alcoves—can also be reconfigured according to need. During active care, these surfaces hold essential items. During vigil, they become spaces for ritual objects, photographs, or tokens of memory. After death, these surfaces may be rearranged to support family reflection, photography, or ceremonial closure. The room's architecture anticipates these shifts without requiring physical intervention.

Child-centered design complements flexibility by reducing emotional and sensory stress. Soft floor mats, low storage, and activity zones allow children to engage in a meaningful but contained way. This design minimizes disruption while acknowledging that children are part of the grieving process, allowing families to remain fully present.

Flexibility in sightlines ensures privacy and dignity. Movable screens, partitions, and furniture placement allow the patient to remain shielded from external views while still permitting family observation and staff access. This dynamic visibility reinforces autonomy and emotional comfort.

Environmental control must adapt to multiple users. Adjustable temperature zones, quiet air circulation, and natural ventilation ensure comfort for patients, staff, and families simultaneously. These features allow the room to be tailored according to the intensity of the ritual, the number of occupants, or the patient's medical condition.

Safety remains integral in flexible design. Movable furniture must be lightweight yet stable, partitions must not obstruct emergency access, and flooring must accommodate both high-traffic family activity and clinical movement. Balancing adaptability with safety ensures that the room remains a supportive environment for all users.

Ultimately, a flexible and adaptable hospice room acknowledges the unpredictable nature of death and human emotion. By designing movable furniture, layered lighting, adaptive acoustics, and multifunctional surfaces, the room becomes capable of supporting every conceivable scenario—from small private vigils to extended family ceremonies, from rapid crises to extended end-of-life reflections.

Flexibility empowers families and staff alike. Families can perform rituals, gather, grieve, and create memory without obstruction, while staff can provide care efficiently and respectfully. The room thus becomes a mediator, a container, and a participant in the profound, multilayered process of dying, ensuring that every end-of-life experience is honored in both function and emotional resonance.

Hospice environments are more than architectural constructs; they are ecological participants in the emotional and physical experience of dying. Integrating the natural world into hospice design transforms a room from a static clinical space into a living, responsive environment. Patients, families, and staff experience profound psychological benefits when views, materials, and sensory cues echo the rhythms of the natural world.

A central principle is the view to nature. Even a simple window overlooking a tree, garden, or sky can reduce anxiety, lower perceived pain, and improve mood. Patients whose line of sight extends to natural forms experience measurable reductions in stress and agitation. The architecture frames these views intentionally: Windows are positioned at eye level from the bed, free of obstructions, and oriented to maximize changing light and shadow patterns across the day.

Natural textures inside the room extend the calming effect. Wooden finishes, stone surfaces, woven fabrics, and ceramic accents evoke the tactile qualities of the outdoors. These materials create a sense of groundedness and connection to life cycles beyond the room itself. The hand on a warm wooden table or the soft weave of a cotton blanket can evoke an emotional stability that sterile surfaces cannot replicate.

Plants and living elements are powerful co-designers. Small potted plants, vertical greenery, or contained moss arrangements introduce subtle movement, color, and scent. They act as living companions, reminding families and patients of growth, continuity, and resilience. Low-maintenance and hypoallergenic species are preferred to ensure health and avoid disruptions to care routines.

Water elements—miniature fountains, tabletop trickling streams, or even the visual presence of a nearby pond—contribute auditory and visual calm. The sound of moving water can mask unwanted mechanical or human noise, providing a subtle, meditative backdrop to vigil hours. Patients report sensations of relaxation when listening to soft water sounds, which also reinforce temporal continuity because flowing water never stops.

The room's design should integrate the weather as an emotional companion. Rain patterns, snow, wind, and sunlight are framed by windows and shaded by architectural elements such as louvers or translucent screens. The patterns of light and shadow created by weather changes act as natural timekeepers, supporting orientation while offering subtle emotional modulation. Families often report comfort in watching seasonal changes, linking the patient's final days to the enduring cycles of nature.

Outdoor sound pathways extend the connection to nature without intruding. Carefully designed acoustic openings allow birdsong, rustling leaves, or distant water sounds to enter the room. Acoustic dampening ensures that these sounds are subtle and controlled, complementing rather than overwhelming the human and mechanical noises inherent to care. This integration reinforces a sense of life continuing outside the walls while maintaining sanctuary within.

Natural light itself is a co-designer. Skylights, clerestory windows, and filtered glazing introduce a spectrum of light and warmth that artificial systems cannot fully replicate. The changing intensity, angle, and color of sunlight mark the passage of hours and support circadian rhythms, enhancing comfort, sleep quality, and emotional orientation for both patients and families.

Seasonal awareness enhances the emotional arc of care. Observing early morning frost, spring blooms, summer sun, or autumn leaves provides a symbolic narrative of life's cycles. Staff and families often incorporate these observations into vigil rituals, storytelling, and memory-making, connecting the patient's journey to a broader temporal continuum.

Even small potted herbs or aromatic plants contribute sensory engagement. Smells of lavender, mint, or rosemary evoke memory, calm, and identity. Families can participate in these interactions, touching leaves, crushing herbs, or rearranging plants, further linking the room to life, growth, and tactile experience.

Architectural framing of views is intentional and symbolic. Window placement, depth of sills, and subtle shading guide the observer to notice movement, light, or color. Patients can track the shifting sky or watch a bird's flight path, creating a quiet dialogue between human presence and the surrounding natural world.

Interior plant arrangements may also serve as ritual anchors. Families often place small mementos or photos near living elements, linking the symbolic vibrancy of nature to the memory and identity of the patient. In this way, plants act as both living companions and emotional facilitators.

Water access within the room supports ritual as well as relaxation. A small fountain may be used to mask noise during meditation, or a basin may be gently used in washing rituals, linking tactile, visual, and auditory cues to caregiving sequences. The symbolic flow of water mirrors the flow of life, reinforcing subtle emotional literacy.

Natural ventilation supports both comfort and psychological well-being. Opening a window or allowing a gentle breeze to pass through the room can signal transitions, provide subtle olfactory stimulation, and maintain air quality. Families often interpret these shifts as a gentle "breathing" of the room, aligning physical and emotional states.

The integration of flora, fauna, and light patterns must be culturally and spiritually sensitive. Some traditions value the presence of living elements as sacred, whereas others may require minimal intervention. Flexibility in placement, variety, and control allows customization according to beliefs while maintaining the integrity of the therapeutic environment.

Material choices extend the narrative of nature indoors. Textured woods, stone countertops, ceramic vessels, and natural fibers signal permanence and continuity, echoing natural cycles. These choices reinforce the idea that life and care exist within broader ecological and temporal frameworks, even at the end of life.

Temporal design and natural cues work in concert. Sunrise and sunset framed through windows, changing foliage patterns, and subtle seasonal shifts in light all structure the emotional day, providing families and staff with implicit guidance on rhythm and ritual. These cues gently remind observers of continuity, impermanence, and the natural arc of life.

Even the smallest view of the sky or garden may evoke profound emotional shifts. Patients and families often experience calm, reflection, or release when noticing a bird landing nearby, raindrops forming patterns on glass, or a shaft of sunlight crossing the room. The natural world becomes a silent participant, a co-designer shaping emotional experience without words.

Finally, the natural world operates as both metaphor and facilitator. Just as daylight signals progression, plants embody resilience, and water reminds of continuity, the architecture of the hospice room collaborates with nature to structure emotion, ritual, and memory. It is a co-designer that allows every participant—patient, family, and staff—to experience presence, comfort, and meaning simultaneously.

The hospice room of the future is imagined not merely as a space for dying but as an active participant in the orchestration of comfort, presence, and emotional attunement. Here, architecture itself becomes a silent caregiver, facilitating human interaction, ritual, and memory in ways that are simultaneously subtle and profound. Each element is deliberately chosen to support patients, families, and staff, ensuring that the environment communicates dignity, peace, and respect without the intrusion of overt instruction or clinical rigidity.

Biophilic design serves as a foundational principle, embedded into every aspect of the room rather than appended as a luxury. Natural materials, filtered daylight, indoor greenery, water features, and gentle soundscapes are not aesthetic flourishes—they are scientifically supported interventions that reduce stress, regulate circadian rhythms, and encourage reflection and memory-making. Every sensory element is curated to foster an emotional equilibrium that complements both care routines and vigil practices.

Designing around ritual rather than purely clinical function marks a transformative shift. The placement of beds, chairs, tables, and memory surfaces anticipates the flow of care and the sequences of human interaction. Bedside rituals, handholding, and the creation of memory altars shape the use of space, allowing architecture to guide movement and attention with a gentle, intuitive authority. Families and caregivers unconsciously navigate the room in patterns that honor both life and transition, without requiring explicit instructions.

Cultural multiplicity is embedded at the conceptual stage. Flexible room configurations, adjustable furniture, and modular surfaces ensure that families of all faiths and traditions can adapt the room to their practices. Whether performing prayer circles, quiet chanting, silent reflection, or musical rituals, the space accommodates diverse needs seamlessly. Design choices honor multiple traditions without privileging one over another, reinforcing the universality of compassion.

Technology operates invisibly but effectively, supporting care while remaining unobtrusive. Automated lighting, climate control, sound masking, and discreet monitoring systems function in the background, maintaining both patient comfort and family privacy. These technologies dissolve into the environment rather than dominating it, allowing the human experience to remain central and unmediated.[3]

The hospice room becomes a caregiver in its own right. Sightlines, spatial configuration, and tactile surfaces communicate permission and safety. A chair by the window invites reflection, a shelf encourages memory-making, and acoustic design allows whispered conversations and prayers to be contained and protected. Every architectural element mediates behavior and emotion, enabling the room to silently participate in care.

Flexibility is a core design principle. Movable furniture, adjustable lighting, and multiuse surfaces allow the room to accommodate unforeseen circumstances, whether a sudden influx of family, extended vigils, or emergent clinical needs. The room is never static; it transforms to meet the emotional, spiritual, and practical demands of the people within it, providing continuity without rigidity.

Spatial clarity and emotional predictability are intertwined. Families navigate without fear of obstacles, staff can access tools efficiently, and patients are never confronted abruptly with machinery or chaotic sightlines. The layout balances privacy, efficiency, and emotional safety, creating an environment that is orderly yet deeply human-centered.

Material honesty reinforces the room's emotional and aesthetic integrity. Woods, stone, ceramics, and natural fibers age gracefully, gaining patina and reinforcing the room's narrative as a repository of memory. Surfaces invite touch, provide grounding, and offer a subtle emotional rhythm, encouraging caregivers and families to interact with space as well as each other.

Natural light is choreographed with precision. Skylights, clerestory windows, and filtered glazing ensure that daylight is never harsh or disorienting. Light patterns shift with the time of day, providing both orientation and emotional modulation. Sunlight entering a room is never static; its movement signals the rhythm of the day, subtly guiding families and staff through ritual, reflection, and care cycles.

Sound is similarly curated. Gentle water features, ambient birdsong, and filtered outdoor sounds provide a calming backdrop. Acoustic zoning ensures that overlapping needs—quiet conversation, clinical interventions, and vigil rituals—coexist without interference. The room orchestrates an aural environment that is supportive and flexible, yet never intrusive, reinforcing calm, focus, and presence.

Memory surfaces are central to emotional continuity. Shelves, tables, and alcoves hold personal objects, photographs, or ritual items in a way that is flexible and temporary. These surfaces support grieving and reflection, allowing families to create narratives, mark presence, and celebrate identity without cluttering or overwhelming the room.

Temporal cues are integrated holistically. Sunrise, sunset, shadow patterns, and seasonal light shifts help structure the day without the need for clocks. Families perceive time intuitively, allowing moments of presence, reflection, and vigil to be shaped by natural rhythms. This design principle transforms the perception of time, making the room a co-participant in life's final stages.

Ergonomics are designed around human dignity. Beds, chairs, and access points prioritize comfort and mobility, while anticipating multigenerational use. Children, adult caregivers, and elderly relatives all find the space accessible, safe, and supportive, allowing the emotional needs of the family to take precedence over mere functionality.

Cultural adaptation is embedded into flexibility. Movable partitions, adjustable furniture, and configurable surfaces allow families to conduct rituals authentically, while maintaining safety and accessibility. The room accommodates religious, spiritual, and cultural practices without requiring compromise, fostering inclusion and respect.

Integration of memory surfaces, light, and acoustics reinforces the emotional tone. A bedside lamp may cast a gentle glow over a curated collection of personal objects, while sound masking ensures intimate conversations are contained. Each element functions synergistically, supporting both ritual and emotional presence.

The room acts as a vessel for presence and transition. It holds the emotional weight of caregiving, vigil, and farewell, while creating pathways for reflection, release, and continuity. Pause zones, contemplative corners, and memory surfaces provide space for individual and collective engagement with the dying process.

Biophilic integration, material warmth, spatial clarity, and ritual flexibility converge to create resilient architecture. The room adapts to unpredictable care needs, supports diverse traditions, and maintains emotional integrity even in moments of profound grief or sudden change. The design becomes simultaneously pragmatic, humane, and spiritually attuned.

Sustainability reinforces both environmental and emotional ethics. Materials are renewable, energy systems efficient, and water features recirculated. Nature is a guiding principle, both practically and symbolically, reinforcing the room's alignment with the rhythms of life and death.

Ultimately, the hospice room becomes a sacred contemporary space. It functions as a team member, silently supporting every participant—patients, families, and staff—through gestures of presence, memory, and dignity. Architecture, nature, and ritual converge to create an environment in which every object, surface, and view contributes to comfort, reflection, and meaning.

7

Soundscapes and Acoustic Design

The absence of sound is rarely neutral. In hospice spaces, silence is not merely the absence of noise but a carefully orchestrated element of design, a medium through which calm, reflection, and emotional safety are conveyed. Physiologically, persistent noise activates the sympathetic nervous system, elevating cortisol and heart rate, and increasing agitation in patients nearing the end of life. In contrast, intentional quiet allows the parasympathetic system to regain balance, fostering relaxation and mental clarity.[1]

For patients with dementia or terminal agitation, noise can be particularly destabilizing. Sudden sounds—clanging carts, slamming doors, and mechanical beeps—can trigger confusion, fear, and even delirium. Architectural interventions, such as the installation of double-glazed windows, acoustic ceiling tiles, and sound-absorbing wall panels, mitigate these intrusions, creating a sanctuary where the mind can rest even when the body is frail.[2]

Carpeted surfaces, although often avoided in hospitals for infection control, are selectively used in hospice rooms to soften footsteps and absorb incidental noise. Modern cleaning protocols, including antimicrobial treatments, allow carpeting to be both hygienic and emotionally supportive. Even minor choices, such as the type of door seal or the padding under furniture, contribute to the overall acoustic envelope of a room.

Sound is also intimately tied to perception of safety. In a noisy environment, patients may experience heightened vigilance or fear, feeling that they must anticipate every sound. A quiet space allows for the suspension of this hyperawareness, permitting families to sit beside a loved one without intrusive distractions. The psychological benefit of this cannot be overstated: Peace of mind for the patient is mirrored in the emotional ease of the family.

One comparative case study involved two hospice rooms designed for identical levels of care. The first room, built in a typical hospital style, reflected hard surfaces, exposed ducts, and a lack of acoustic treatments. Families reported frequent disturbances and noted that they felt "on edge" throughout visits. In contrast, a room with acoustically treated walls, quiet mechanical systems, and soft textiles allowed families to stay for hours without fatigue or tension. Patients appeared calmer, with measurable reductions in heart rate and agitation episodes.[3]

The design of silence requires attention not only to the built environment but also to human behavior. Staff are trained to move quietly, roll carts softly, and speak in modulated tones during vigil hours. These behavioral protocols complement architectural interventions, reinforcing the room's purpose as a space of reflection and care. Families quickly notice these subtle cues, often describing the experience as entering a "different world" from the busy corridors outside.

Research in environmental psychology supports these findings, showing that reduced sound levels in care settings correlate with improved patient outcomes, including decreased agitation, fewer medication interventions, and enhanced sleep quality.[4] For hospice care, the stakes are emotional as much as physical: Calm facilitates presence, which is the essence of end-of-life care.

Silence also allows the emotional content of speech to be fully appreciated. In rooms in which noise dominates, whispered prayers, last conversations, or quiet song may be drowned out or feel muted. In intentionally quiet rooms, these sounds become carriers of meaning. Families recount moments when a simple whispered memory or prayer, heard clearly in the soft environment, became a pivotal part of their emotional processing.

The acoustic environment can influence circadian rhythms, even in patients who are bedridden. Nighttime silence, combined with dimmed lighting, supports natural sleep–wake cycles, reducing confusion and sundowning behaviors in patients with cognitive decline. The synchronization of auditory and visual cues creates an integrated temporal framework that both staff and families intuitively follow.

Even routine interventions, such as clinical monitoring or repositioning a patient, are experienced differently in quiet spaces. A gentle touch accompanied by the absence of mechanical clatter reassures patients that care is attentive but not intrusive. Families often comment on how the quiet magnifies these small gestures, making them feel deeply significant.

A narrative shared by a hospice family illustrates this point: A daughter described sitting beside her father in a room in which the only sound was the soft hum of filtered ventilation. She noticed that the silence made her father's breathing the most present element, each inhalation and exhalation a rhythm to anchor the vigil. The absence of extraneous sound allowed her to "be fully there" in ways that hospital visits never permitted.

Acoustic design also extends to intentional sound masking. Low-level ambient noise—such as soft white noise or filtered nature sounds—can create a buffer that prevents intrusive hallway sounds from entering the room. This technique maintains the perception of silence while protecting the delicate emotional atmosphere.

Importantly, silence is not uniform; it is shaped into zones of auditory experience. Micro-zones within a room—such as the bedside, the family chair, and staff alcoves—allow for different levels of sound intensity. The patient zone may be closest to absolute quiet, whereas the family chair accommodates whispered conversation or soft music. Staff alcoves may support clinical communication without intruding on the emotional space.

Acoustic materials themselves carry symbolic weight. Soft textiles, wooden surfaces, and muted wall finishes communicate care through sensory perception. The patina of wood, for example, absorbs sound while providing a visual reminder of warmth and human touch. Families often comment on the subtle reassurance of these textures, which suggest that the space was intentionally designed for care rather than merely function.

In addition to physical materials, the spatial arrangement of objects can affect sound behavior. Bookshelves, upholstered furniture, and strategically placed curtains scatter sound reflections, preventing harsh echoes. Even small interventions, such as hanging textile panels or using wall-mounted art with soft backing, contribute to the overall acoustic quality.

Acoustic design also plays a role in ritual and transition. The moment a patient passes is often marked by intentional silence, allowing families to recognize the shift without abrupt intrusion. Staff may dim lights and pause their own movements, creating a shared sensory experience in which the absence of sound communicates respect and closure.

Anecdotal evidence suggests that silence fosters intergenerational connection. Children visiting a hospice room may notice that the quiet encourages gentle speech, leaning close to hold hands, and observing the rhythm of a dying person's breath. In this way, acoustic design subtly shapes behavior, reinforcing care and intimacy.

From a design perspective, silence is as much about what is removed as what is included. Eliminating harsh mechanical sounds, minimizing echo, and creating buffer zones are as important as introducing any intentional sound. The interplay between absence and presence of sound defines the emotional architecture of the room.

In planning new hospice spaces, architects increasingly collaborate with acoustic consultants, behavioral psychologists, and experienced hospice staff. This interdisciplinary approach ensures that the principles of quiet are integrated into construction, finishing materials, and operational protocols, rather than being an afterthought.

Finally, silence serves as a foundation for all other sensory interventions. It enhances light, color, texture, and ritual by providing a receptive environment. Without the carefully considered orchestration of quiet, other design elements risk being overlooked or diluted. In this way, the science of silence becomes the scaffold upon which emotional hospice care is constructed.

Environmental soundscapes in hospice care extend the concept of silence by layering intentional auditory cues that enhance emotional well-being. Natural sounds—such as the gentle burble of water, the rustle of leaves, or distant bird calls—act as anchors, grounding patients and families in the present while subtly signaling the passage of time. The careful integration of these sounds transforms a room from a passive container into an active participant in care.

Water is one of the most potent auditory tools in hospice environments. The rhythmic trickle of a small indoor fountain or the distant sound of a protected outdoor water feature creates a continuous, soft auditory backdrop. This gentle murmur functions as a low-level white noise, masking disruptive mechanical sounds while simultaneously offering a comforting and meditative presence. For patients experiencing anxiety, terminal restlessness, or disorientation, the steady rhythm of flowing water provides a sensory tether, helping regulate breathing and emotional state.[5]

Wind chimes, often hung near windows or sheltered outdoor courtyards, serve as dynamic markers of wind, season, and movement. Their soft, unpredictable tones introduce a subtle liveliness to the environment without overwhelming the senses. Families frequently report that the sound of chimes evokes memories of home gardens or natural settings, linking the hospice environment to familiar and reassuring places. The gentle unpredictability of these sounds mirrors the natural variability of life, providing both comfort and reflection.

Birdsong, carefully introduced either through open windows in protected outdoor areas or via low-volume sound systems, has been shown to reduce stress and promote positive emotional states. Morning bird calls, in particular, provide an intuitive cue for the start of the day, reinforcing circadian rhythms without the clinical harshness of alarms. Families often note that hearing birdsong during vigil hours encourages quiet reflection, as the natural soundscape fosters a contemplative mood.[6]

The auditory integration of nature can be achieved through indoor–outdoor spatial design. Rooms with open views to protected gardens or courtyards allow patients and families to experience environmental sounds directly, enhancing orientation and the perception of connection to the broader world. Architectural elements, such as window placement, screened porches, or sound-permeable walls, allow nature's rhythms to enter the hospice space without compromising safety or privacy.

Temporal variation in sound is also essential. Seasonal changes, daily fluctuations, and weather-driven differences create a natural rhythm within the hospice environment. The sound of rain tapping softly against windows during an afternoon vigil can evoke a reflective mood, whereas morning bird calls can gently energize staff and family members. Designing spaces that accommodate these temporal variations allows the environment to function as a subtle guide to daily and seasonal cycles.

Case studies underscore the power of environmental soundscapes. One patient, experiencing increasing agitation during the final week of life, became noticeably calmer when positioned near a small indoor fountain whose soft trickle was audible but not intrusive. Morning visits by family coincided with the sounds of nearby birds in a sheltered courtyard. Staff reported that the patient's breathing stabilized and periods of restlessness decreased during these hours, highlighting the direct effect of the natural sound environment on physiological and emotional states.

Staff observations further illustrate the impact. During family gatherings, nurses noted that the sound of water and wind created an almost sacred atmosphere in which whispered conversations, prayers, and story-sharing were naturally paced and softened. Families described feeling as though the room itself "listened" and "participated," a perception reinforced by the presence of unobtrusive, calming natural sounds.

Soundscapes also function as emotional transitions. During vigil hours, the shift from daytime activity to evening quiet can be enhanced with subtle environmental cues: the gentle rustling of trees as the breeze picks up, or the fading call of birds as dusk approaches. These auditory signals reinforce the natural rhythm of the day and guide both staff and families intuitively, without verbal instruction or mechanical alarms.

From a design perspective, the positioning of sound elements is crucial. Water features should be placed where their sound carries softly across the room without overwhelming speech or ritual activities. Wind chimes or vegetation should be positioned to maximize gentle resonance while avoiding sharp or sudden sounds that may startle patients. This attention to placement ensures that environmental soundscape integration supports the emotional arc of care rather than disrupting it.

Acoustic engineering complements environmental sound design. Sound absorption and diffusion materials help balance natural sounds, ensuring that the auditory environment remains soft and comforting. Carpets, wall panels, and upholstered surfaces reduce echo and prevent unintended amplification, creating a coherent and immersive experience. The interplay between environmental sounds and controlled acoustics enhances perception of calm, continuity, and presence.

Narrative accounts frequently highlight the symbolic dimensions of sound. One family described the morning they realized the wind chimes were moving in harmony with their loved one's slow, rhythmic breathing. The natural cadence of the room became an emotional metaphor for life and transition, reinforcing the sacred quality of vigil hours.

Soundscapes also support multisensory integration. Paired with gentle lighting, tactile materials, and curated objects, natural sounds reinforce the emotional resonance of the space. A leaf-strewn garden visible through a window, the soft trickle of water, and the scent of fresh flowers combine to create a holistic, emotionally stabilizing environment that supports reflection and ritual.

Environmental sounds can also act as cues for family behavior. In some cases, soft water or wind sounds encourage quiet conversation, gentle movement, or attentive observation, subtly shaping the rhythm of human activity without explicit instruction. Families often report that these sounds reduce anxiety and create a sense of emotional containment, allowing them to focus on presence rather than procedural care.

During high-intensity periods, such as the arrival of multiple visitors or the preparation for a patient's passing, natural soundscapes provide continuity and emotional ballast. They create a background rhythm that anchors attention, reduces overstimulation, and reinforces the sacredness of the moment.

Considerations of cultural sensitivity are also important. Different families may associate specific natural sounds with distinct emotional or spiritual meanings. Design should allow for flexibility, such as providing options to emphasize or mute certain sound sources according to family preference. This ensures that soundscapes are inclusive and supportive rather than prescriptive.

Technology can enhance environmental soundscapes without compromising authenticity. Discreetly placed speakers can introduce subtle bird calls or flowing water in rooms in which direct exposure to outdoor environments is limited. Volume, timing, and tonal quality are carefully controlled to preserve emotional balance and avoid intrusiveness.

Staff training is essential for maximizing the benefits of environmental sound. Caregivers learn to position patients in ways that optimize exposure to calming natural sounds and to coordinate activity schedules around auditory cues. Families can also be educated about how to interact with and respect these subtle environmental elements, reinforcing the shared nature of care.

Finally, environmental soundscapes reinforce the broader philosophy of hospice as a human-centered, multisensory experience. They remind caregivers, families, and designers alike that the room itself is active in emotional support, subtly guiding behavior, marking time, and creating a sacred container for the final stages of life. The orchestration of nature's sounds transforms space into a living, breathing partner in the work of care.

The human voice is one of the most intimate and emotionally resonant elements in hospice care, functioning as both a bridge and a container for presence, memory, and ritual. Whispered conversations, prayers, storytelling, and singing create a sound layer distinct from the environmental or mechanical sounds of the hospice room, serving simultaneously as guidance, comfort, and continuity. Unlike music or ambient sound, the human voice carries relational significance, immediately connecting patients, families, and staff to one another.

The placement of furniture and seating profoundly affects how voice travels and is perceived in a hospice room. Chairs positioned near the bedside, angled slightly toward the patient, create a natural acoustic geometry that enhances projection without requiring amplification. Soft textiles, upholstered surfaces, and strategically placed rugs prevent harsh echoes, allowing whispers and quiet singing to be heard clearly while maintaining intimacy. In this way, spatial design functions as a silent collaborator in vocal communication.

Volume and timbre are critical in voice-mediated care. A quiet, steady tone can reassure a patient and signal safety, whereas sudden loudness can induce anxiety or agitation. Care teams often adopt voice modulation protocols: soft cadence, measured pauses, and gentle projection that emphasize presence over instruction. Families often unconsciously mimic these patterns, creating a shared auditory language that reinforces calm and connection.

Narratives shared by families illustrate the power of the human voice. One daughter described reading aloud from her mother's favorite poetry book each evening. The act of whispering each line, pausing to let her mother respond through small gestures or sighs, became a ritual that transformed the room into a sacred space. The quiet intimacy allowed other family members to enter the room respectfully, guided by the pace and tone of the reading.

Storytelling functions as both legacy and comfort. Families recount memories, recite letters, or share private jokes as a way to maintain relational continuity and affirm identity. The spatial positioning of chairs and the patient's bed often dictates how voices carry. A bedside chair angled toward the patient and near the window not only enhances projection but also situates the speaker in the patient's visual field, reinforcing a sense of presence.

Singing, whether formal or improvised, introduces a harmonic dimension that enhances emotional resonance. Hymns, lullabies, or culturally significant songs are particularly effective when voice carries naturally through the space, supported by soft acoustic surfaces. Families report that singing during vigil hours can calm restlessness, ease transitions between activity and quiet, and create shared moments of reflection and connection.

The cadence of the human voice, like music, can mirror physiological rhythms. Slow, measured speech tends to lower heart rate and respiratory effort in patients, providing a gentle counterpoint to anxiety or discomfort. Quick, irregular speech, conversely, can exacerbate distress. Staff are trained to observe patient response and adjust tone and pace accordingly, reinforcing a feedback loop in which the room's acoustic and emotional environment aligns with human needs.

Voice as ritual is also spatially mediated. During nighttime vigils, whispered conversations allow families to share memories and prayers without disturbing other patients or staff. These whispered exchanges become part of the ritual of presence, creating a layered auditory environment in which the room itself seems to participate. Architectural design supports this by controlling sound reflection, minimizing corridors' intrusion, and using soft partitions to allow multiple simultaneous conversations.

Staff reflections underscore the intentionality required in voice use. Nurses, chaplains, and volunteers often pause mid-task to modulate their speech, choosing words and delivery that acknowledge both patient autonomy and family emotion. Even routine updates about care, delivered with a gentle tone and careful pacing, contribute to the room's emotional temperature. The human voice, in this context, is as much a tool of architecture as it is a relational medium.

Whispered rituals have measurable psychological effects. In patients with terminal agitation or delirium, staff note that soft, predictable voice patterns reduce agitation episodes and support restful breathing. Families also report that coordinated voice use during shared storytelling fosters a sense of co-presence, reinforcing the feeling that they are not merely observers but participants in the patient's journey.

The timing of vocal interventions matters. Morning readings, soft songs at dusk, and whispered prayers during vigil hours create a temporal structure that mirrors natural circadian rhythms. The room's acoustics amplify this effect: Sound travels predictably, enabling all occupants to orient themselves to ritual without explicit instruction. Over time, these vocal cues become embedded in the collective memory of the space.

Acoustic geometry also supports emotional layering. A small alcove for staff or family observers allows multiple voices to coexist without interference. A storyteller may sit near the patient, while another family member contributes from a secondary position. The room, through careful spatial and acoustic design, accommodates overlapping vocal expressions without generating chaos or confusion.

Cultural and spiritual traditions influence voice use. Chanting, prayer, or call-and-response patterns are often incorporated into care routines. The architecture of the room can amplify or soften these expressions, ensuring that sound enhances rather than overwhelms. Families report that when the room "resonates" with culturally meaningful vocal patterns, it strengthens the sense of sacredness and shared purpose.

Voice is intimately linked to tactile and visual engagement. Whispered readings paired with handholding, gentle touch, or eye contact deepen the emotional effect. Families describe these multisensory interactions as profoundly grounding, with the human voice serving as the connective thread that binds touch, presence, and ritual together.

Even staff-to-staff communication benefits from intentional voice use. Quiet, respectful speech allows coordination of care without disrupting patient or family engagement. During high-intensity periods, such as end-of-life transitions, staff may adopt a shared code of tone and volume, maintaining operational efficiency while preserving the sanctuary of the room.

Environmental integration enhances voice perception. Soft furnishings, acoustic panels, and carefully chosen flooring materials ensure that whispers travel clearly to the intended listener without reverberating harshly. This creates a subtle layering of sound in which both intended and ambient voices contribute to the overall emotional ecosystem.

Family stories often highlight the emotional layering achieved through voice. One granddaughter recounted telling a beloved story from childhood while other family members quietly contributed memories. The room absorbed these voices, and the patient's faint responses—gestures, eye movements, or sighs—amplified their significance. The space itself seemed to participate in the storytelling, absorbing and reflecting the collective emotional intent.

Voice also functions as a temporal guide. Families and staff often unconsciously adjust the pace of conversation based on patient cues, sunlight, or environmental sounds. A gentle murmur of wind through trees outside can inspire a soft cadence, reinforcing the interconnectedness of voice, environment, and ritual.

Finally, the human voice serves as a bridge between the tangible and the intangible. Whispered words, recited memories, and softly sung songs convey love, presence, and care in ways that architectural elements alone cannot. Yet, when integrated with spatial design, acoustic treatment, and environmental soundscapes, voice becomes a component of the room's architecture itself—a dynamic instrument of comfort, ritual, and continuity.

Hospice spaces exist at the intersection of comfort and functionality. While the room's architecture, light, and environmental soundscapes create emotional stability, intrusive noise can undermine these carefully curated elements. Mechanical sounds—alarms, hallway traffic, heating, ventilation, and air-conditioning (HVAC) hums, and equipment wheels—intervene in delicate emotional and physiological states, disrupting sleep, focus, and the continuity of rituals. Recognizing and controlling these sounds is therefore a foundational principle of compassionate design.

Noise management begins with understanding its physiological and psychological impact. Studies show that sudden or persistent high-decibel sounds trigger stress hormone release; elevate heart rate; and can exacerbate terminal agitation, delirium, or restlessness. Even subtle disruptions—such as the echo of a hallway trolley or a distant alarm—can momentarily disorient patients, particularly those with cognitive decline or sensory sensitivity. Families, too, are affected, often experiencing heightened anxiety when the environment feels unpredictable or jarring.

Clinical workflows intersect with acoustic reality. Nurses and aides frequently navigate multiple patients, administer medications, and manage equipment, all while striving to maintain a quiet and reassuring presence. Strategic noise control requires both environmental solutions and behavior protocols. Physical interventions—such as acoustic panels, carpeting, soft-closing doors, and rubberized caster wheels—mitigate mechanical and foot traffic noise, ensuring that daily operational sounds remain unobtrusive.

Staff behaviors are equally significant. Rolling carts must be maneuvered slowly, doors closed with intentional softness, and conversations kept to low volumes. Even small adjustments, such as using felt pads under furniture legs or lowering the tone of announcements over the public address system, cumulatively reduce sound intrusion. Staff training emphasizes that these behaviors are not merely etiquette but an integral component of therapeutic design.

White noise or sound-masking systems are sometimes employed in strategic locations to preserve privacy. A low-level hum, designed to blend with environmental sounds, can mask sudden noises without adding cognitive burden. These systems are especially valuable in units in which multiple rooms share walls or where HVAC systems produce intermittent, unavoidable sounds. White noise effectively creates an acoustic buffer, allowing patients and families to maintain focus on presence and ritual rather than being startled by distant activity.

The difference between a carefully managed room and a standard clinical environment is stark. In one comparative case, two hospice rooms housed patients with similar care needs and routines. In the first room, soft furnishings, acoustic panels, and attentive staff protocols minimized background noise. In the second, linoleum floors, open doors, and untreated ceilings allowed equipment, foot traffic, and hallway noise to intrude. Families in the first room reported a sense of peace and safety; those in the second described intermittent anxiety and distraction, even during otherwise quiet hours.

Hallway traffic is a common source of auditory disruption. Patients often perceive distant conversations or passing footsteps as closer than they are, particularly when rooms lack sound-absorbing finishes. Designing buffer zones—such as recessed alcoves, double doors, or acoustic corridors—reduces the transmission of these sounds. Strategic placement of staff workstations away from patient rooms further minimizes inadvertent noise intrusion, preserving the sanctity of vigil hours.

Alarms present a unique challenge. Although critical for patient safety, they can be emotionally jarring. Modern hospice units often employ systems that allow selective alarm routing to staff pagers rather than audible hallway alerts. This approach ensures rapid clinical response while minimizing patient and family exposure to sudden, high-decibel noises.

HVAC systems are another subtle but significant factor. Airflow noise, temperature fluctuation hums, or mechanical rattling can intrude into the room's soundscape. Careful specification of low-noise fans, vibration isolation mounts, and duct design reduces these unintended sounds. Environmental engineers often collaborate with interior designers to achieve both thermal comfort and acoustic serenity.

Even seemingly minor sounds—the clatter of a dropped instrument, the squeak of a chair, or the click of medical devices—can disrupt the fragile emotional ecosystem of a hospice room. Protocols that encourage mindfulness in motion, slower handling of equipment, and anticipatory movement patterns are essential. These behaviors are as much a part of care as administering medications, underscoring the integration of sound awareness into daily practice.

Families frequently comment on the emotional relief experienced in rooms with intentional noise control. The absence of intrusive sound allows whispered stories, prayers, or singing to resonate fully. Subtle differences in sound levels alter perceived intimacy: A low, constant hum of machinery may create anxiety, whereas a quiet, acoustically controlled environment fosters reflection and presence.

The psychological impact of controlled noise is particularly evident during final hours. Vigil hours, when families are present for prolonged periods, are especially sensitive to auditory intrusions. Staff describe that even minimal background noise can break emotional concentration, interrupting handholding rituals or whispered storytelling. Conversely, when sound is carefully managed, families report that they feel held by the space itself, a subtle reinforcement of safety and care.

Spatial design also mediates acoustic exposure. Rooms positioned away from high-traffic corridors, elevators, and nursing stations naturally experience fewer disturbances. Windows with double-glazing or acoustic coatings minimize external street or garden noise. The combination of spatial, material, and behavioral strategies transforms what might otherwise be a chaotic auditory environment into a sanctuary of calm.

Case narratives reveal cumulative effects. In one hospice, two neighboring rooms housed patients with similar illness severity. Patients in the room with soft flooring, acoustic wall panels, and who had staff trained in noise mindfulness experienced fewer agitation events and more restful sleep, and higher family satisfaction scores were reported for this room. The comparison highlights that even subtle acoustic interventions—without altering clinical routines—produce measurable differences in care experience.

White noise and sound masking require careful calibration. Too loud, and they compete with voices or environmental sounds, reducing their effectiveness. Too soft, and they fail to mask mechanical intrusion. Successful implementation depends on continuous observation and adjustment, often in real time, by both staff and designers.

Staff reflections also emphasize the relational aspect of noise management. Being attentive to sound is not purely technical; it conveys care, attentiveness, and respect. Families often interpret quiet, deliberate movements and gentle handling of equipment as signs of emotional presence, reinforcing the overall therapeutic environment.

Behavioral routines complement architectural design. Soft shoes, lowered conversations, and staggered movements create a rhythm of care that allows both staff and families to coexist in the room harmoniously. These micro-behaviors are taught through shadowing, mentorship, and deliberate orientation to the hospice's acoustic philosophy.

Noise control intersects with ritual. During body care, final conversations, or readings, even minor mechanical sounds can intrude. Conversely, the absence of such disruptions amplifies the emotional resonance of ritual. Families note that when alarms are routed discreetly, carts are rolled silently, and HVAC noise is minimized, the room itself feels "present" and supportive.

Ultimately, noise control in hospice spaces is more than functional—it is deeply ethical. It signals that emotional experience matters as much as clinical efficiency, and that every design choice, staff behavior, and technological intervention can support or undermine presence, reflection, and ritual. Thoughtful management of intrusive sound honors the patient, the family, and the emotional labor of staff in equal measure.

Sound, when intentionally integrated into hospice spaces, becomes a profound marker of sacred time. In addition to its practical roles in communication or background ambiance, sound can signify transition, presence, and closure. Vigil hours, bedside prayers, or the final moments of life are all enhanced when auditory cues are deliberately designed into the environment. In this way, sound transforms from incidental noise into a vessel for emotional and spiritual resonance.

The start of a vigil is often accompanied by subtle auditory cues. A soft chime, a gentle bell, or the onset of a familiar song can signify that the sacred period of presence has begun. These cues communicate to both staff and families that ordinary time has shifted into a heightened, attentive space of care and reflection.

The patient, attuned to rhythm and pattern, often senses these transitions intuitively, even in the absence of conscious recognition.

Music therapy is a particularly effective modality for marking transitions. Adapted to the patient's cultural, spiritual, and personal preferences, music can soothe agitation, reinforce memory, and create a shared ritual for families. A simple, repetitive melody may become an anchor for collective attention, while a familiar hymn or folk song evokes meaningful life narratives. Selecting adaptive and culturally sensitive music ensures that rituals resonate without alienating any participant.

Low-volume chimes or bell tones are often used to signal transitions subtly. These sounds, when placed strategically within a room or courtyard, communicate ritualistic shifts without interrupting the room's emotional atmosphere. Unlike louder alarms or mechanical signals, soft chimes invite reflection rather than anxiety. Families report that the gentle ringing marks the beginning or end of vigil hours, creating a temporal structure that is both reassuring and meaningful.

Recorded nature cues, such as water flowing, rustling leaves, or distant bird calls, can also function as ritual markers. Timed with circadian rhythms or the unfolding of final care, these sounds remind both patient and family of continuity with the natural world, reinforcing life cycles even in the context of mortality. Architectural features, such as open windows or recessed outdoor sound pathways, allow these cues to blend seamlessly with indoor acoustics.

Families often attach emotional significance to particular songs or sounds during final days. One family associated the patient's favorite piano composition with nightly reading rituals. Over time, hearing this song—even outside the hospice—evoked vivid memories of presence, care, and intimacy. The room, in this sense, not only hosts ritual but also imprints lasting emotional resonance, mediated by carefully curated sound.

Spatial design supports ritualized sound. Alcoves, soft furnishings, and partitioning allow multiple voices, instruments, or chimes to coexist without conflict. The architecture ensures that ritual sounds reach intended listeners without disturbing adjacent rooms or staff operations. Families and staff experience this as a form of acoustic sanctuary, where sacred moments are contained and honored.

The timing and sequence of ritual sounds are also significant. A bedside bell may precede a reading, signaling families to gather, while the fading notes of a song or chime mark the conclusion of a vigil. This temporal choreography helps orient participants, providing a subtle rhythm to emotionally intense moments. Patients often respond unconsciously to these cues, aligning their attention or presence with the ritualized sequence.

Staff play an active role in supporting these auditory rituals. Nurses, chaplains, and volunteers may initiate or conclude sound cues, adjusting volume, tone, or selection based on the emotional state of the patient and family. This requires attentiveness, emotional literacy, and sensitivity to both cultural context and individual preference.

Voice is a central element of ritualized sound. Whispered prayers, storytelling, or song may be integrated into musical or chime-based transitions. Staff guidance ensures that these voices are heard clearly, harmonizing with environmental and technological sound cues. Families often mirror these patterns, creating layered soundscapes that enrich the emotional experience.

Technology can facilitate ritualized sound without disrupting the sanctuary of the room. Hidden speakers, automated timers, or integrated sound systems allow subtle playback of music, nature sounds, or chimes. These systems, when architecturally and operationally designed, dissolve into the background, allowing ritual to unfold organically rather than feeling artificial or intrusive.

Sound as ritual is often linked to spatial orientation. Specific sounds may be associated with defined zones: bedside, reflection corners, or memory surfaces. A chime near the window chair, for instance, may signal the start of a family storytelling session, while gentle music at the bedside marks the moment of intimate presence. Spatially differentiated sound supports predictability and emotional grounding.

Families frequently recount that ritualized sound helps manage grief and anxiety. A carefully timed song or chime offers a cue to pause, reflect, and bear witness, creating a shared emotional rhythm. These cues often persist in memory after the patient has passed, becoming a mnemonic anchor for continued connection and commemoration.

Cultural and spiritual traditions shape the selection and timing of ritual sounds. In Buddhist practice, bells may mark breath cycles or transitions; in Catholic care, hymns may accompany prayer; Indigenous practices may incorporate flute or drum. Architectural flexibility ensures that no tradition is privileged over another while supporting these auditory rituals.

The predictability of ritualized sound fosters psychological safety. Patients and families learn to anticipate auditory cues, reducing anxiety and creating a sense of continuity. Staff report that when rituals are consistently supported by sound, emotional responses are calmer, and transitions—such as repositioning, caregiving, or the final hours—proceed with greater grace.

Sound layering enhances ritual. Whispered narratives, instrumental music, nature recordings, and chimes may coexist, each serving a different emotional or temporal function. The architecture, furnishings, and acoustic treatment ensure these layers complement rather than conflict, reinforcing the integrity of the ritualized environment.

The integration of ritualized sound also supports intergenerational participation. Children, often sensitive to both visual and auditory cues, respond to predictable sound patterns. Soft music, chimes, or whispered storytelling allows them to engage without feeling overwhelmed, providing comfort and inclusion in end-of-life presence.

Staff observations highlight subtle effects of ritualized sound. Even when no family is present, the anticipation of a chime or song encourages reflection and focus. Rooms with integrated auditory rituals are described as "alive but calm," communicating a persistent sense of attentive care.

Sound as ritual reinforces the broader hospice philosophy that every sensory dimension contributes to care. By intentionally orchestrating auditory cues, spaces support dignity, emotional presence, and ritual continuity. Patients, families, and staff experience these moments as profoundly meaningful, demonstrating that architecture and sound together constitute an active participant in end-of-life care.

Finally, the ethical dimension of sound ritual is clear. Deliberate, respectful, culturally sensitive auditory design conveys care, presence, and acknowledgment of life's transitions. By integrating sound into ritual, hospice environments honor both the temporal and spiritual aspects of dying, creating spaces in which memory, love, and closure are audibly embodied.

8

Olfactory Design in Hospice

Scent is one of the most intimate and powerful sensory modalities, deeply intertwined with memory, identity, and emotion. In hospice care, olfactory experiences are more than incidental: They provide continuity, emotional grounding, and a subtle form of presence. Familiar scents, whether drawn from a patient's home, cultural practices, or natural materials, can anchor memory and ritual, allowing both patient and family to inhabit the hospice space in a way that feels emotionally connected and personally significant. By thoughtfully integrating smell into care, hospice environments move beyond functional design into the realm of sensory sanctuary, where each fragrance can evoke memory, comfort, and dignity.

The neurological foundations for olfactory influence are profound. Olfactory receptors connect directly to the limbic system, the part of the brain responsible for emotion and memory. This direct connection explains why a single whiff of lavender, wood smoke, or a family-specific fragrance can evoke vivid memories and strong emotional responses.[1] In end-of-life settings, these scents can reconnect patients with aspects of their identity, past experiences, and life narratives, creating a profound sense of continuity even as the patient approaches death. Families often witness moments in which a familiar aroma evokes recognition or emotional clarity that words alone cannot achieve.

Lavender has been extensively studied for its calming effects.[2] Its subtle aroma reduces anxiety, lowers heart rate, and fosters a sense of stillness. In hospice rooms, controlled diffusion of lavender during vigil hours can create a gentle, comforting atmosphere without overwhelming the patient. However, careful moderation is critical; overuse risks nausea, sensory overstimulation, or aversion, particularly in patients with hypersensitive olfactory perception or respiratory conditions. The strategic use of scent ensures that it functions as a supportive emotional tool rather than a clinical gimmick.

In addition to lavender, other familiar scents—such as vanilla, sandalwood, chamomile, or pine—carry unique emotional resonance. Families often bring items infused with these fragrances: a favorite candle, an old quilt, a sachet of dried herbs, or a familiar soap. These objects act as olfactory bridges to the patient's history, linking hospice care with personal, lived experience. The smells evoke life narratives, evoke comfort, and often provide a stabilizing effect during emotionally intense moments, creating an intimate and home-like environment.

Consider the case of a patient with advanced dementia. When a caregiver brought a favorite home candle with a subtle vanilla scent into the room, the patient, previously agitated and unresponsive, became calm and focused. The patient was able to recognize family members, engage briefly in conversation, and exhibit a sense of emotional presence that had been absent for days. This example illustrates the profound capacity of smell to re-establish connection and identity, even in the final stages of life.

Families frequently report that olfactory experiences provide deeply personal moments of connection. A daughter arranging a small vase of lavender recalled her mother's garden; a son lighting incense brought from home evoked shared journeys and intimate memories. These scent-based rituals allow families to participate actively in caregiving, turning otherwise mundane tasks into gestures of love, remembrance, and presence. The ritualization of smell contributes to emotional closure, shared storytelling, and intergenerational engagement.

Placement and method of scent delivery are crucial. Overhead diffusers, portable oil burners, or lightly scented linens allow subtle dispersion without overwhelming the room. Strategic placement near memory surfaces, bedside tables, or reflection chairs ensures the fragrance enhances ritual rather than becoming intrusive. Portable solutions, such as small sachets or scented cloths, allow families to participate in creating these olfactory moments, fostering a sense of agency in the care environment.

Scent is often integrated with other sensory modalities to strengthen ritual. A lavender-infused washcloth combined with soft lighting, gentle touch, and comforting textiles creates a multilayered experience that reinforces emotional presence. By engaging multiple senses simultaneously, hospice staff help patients maintain cognitive and emotional continuity, allowing families to bear witness to life and memory in a holistic, embodied way.

Cultural sensitivity is central to olfactory design. Fragrances can carry religious, spiritual, or ancestral significance. Frankincense may be integral to Catholic or Orthodox rites, sweetgrass to Indigenous traditions, and jasmine or sandalwood to certain Asian practices. Hospice staff must recognize these traditions, accommodating ritual-specific scents while ensuring that the environment remains inclusive and respectful of all participants. Proper integration prevents the privileging of one cultural narrative over another and allows rituals to remain authentic.

Olfactory experiences often accompany storytelling. Diffusing a patient's favorite scent during family reminiscence can strengthen the emotional resonance of memories. These moments link olfactory and verbal memory, creating lasting mnemonic anchors that persist beyond the patient's death. Families frequently recount that the combination of scent and story evokes more vivid recollections than storytelling alone, illustrating the multisensory nature of memory.

The subtlety of scent is essential. Strong, pervasive aromas can become intrusive or irritating, particularly for patients with sensitive olfactory systems or respiratory vulnerabilities. By calibrating the intensity and timing of scent delivery, hospice spaces preserve olfactory cues as supportive emotional accents, rather than overpowering the room's sensory environment.

Temporal orchestration of scent is important. Certain fragrances may be introduced only during vigil hours or alternating periods to prevent adaptation and sensory desensitization. This rhythm aligns with other hospice temporal strategies, including lighting transitions, acoustic cues, and tactile interventions, ensuring that olfactory moments remain meaningful and emotionally salient.

Scent can also guide staff behavior. Recognizable olfactory cues signal transitions, such as the beginning of vigil or a storytelling session. Staff attuned to these cues may adjust their movement, voice, and attentiveness accordingly, fostering a synchronized, ritualized atmosphere in the room that supports both patients and families.

Memory surfaces—tables, shelves, and micro-altars—serve as focal points for scent-based rituals. Dried flowers, scented cloths, and personal oils can be placed on these surfaces to reinforce the emotional significance of objects. By integrating smell with visual and tactile cues, these arrangements create rich multisensory experiences that enhance presence, reflection, and emotional continuity.

Olfactory design also contributes to perceived comfort. Even when architecture, lighting, and acoustics are optimal, a neutral or sterile smell can evoke a clinical or impersonal atmosphere. Introducing subtle, familiar scents enhances home-likeness, warmth, and emotional security, allowing the hospice room to function as a psychologically safe space.

The timing of scent introduction can mark significant transitional moments. A carefully chosen aroma diffused at the patient's arrival, during rituals, or as death approaches can cue presence, reflection, and closure. Families often describe these scents as inseparable from their memories of care, underscoring the enduring power of olfactory design.

Staff observations indicate that olfactory cues can subtly influence patient behavior. Terminal restlessness, anxiety, or agitation is often mitigated by familiar or calming scents. Patients become more receptive to touch, conversation, and ritual engagement, highlighting scent's dual role as environmental and therapeutic tool.

Architectural considerations support olfactory integration. Ventilation systems, airflow patterns, and material selection influence how scent disperses, lingers, or is absorbed. Natural materials such as wood, linen, and cotton retain subtle aromas, extending the presence of memory-associated scents without compromising air quality or comfort.

Scent rituals extend to families as well. Bringing familiar aromas into the room encourages reflection, storytelling, and shared participation in care. These multisensory experiences strengthen relational bonds, allowing grief, love, and presence to coexist in the hospice environment in ways that are deeply remembered.

Finally, olfactory design in hospice underscores the broader philosophy that all senses contribute to compassionate care. By thoughtfully curating smell as a memory and ritual anchor, hospice environments foster emotional stability, reinforce identity, and support the rituals of presence, storytelling, and farewell. In this way, the hospice room becomes a space in which life, memory, and love persist in subtle, multisensory ways.

Aromatherapy in hospice is more than a decorative or aesthetic choice; it is a deliberate tool for emotional regulation and psychological comfort. Essential oils, herbal infusions, and subtle scent diffusers are employed to create an environment that reduces anxiety, alleviates agitation, and fosters a sense of calm. The use of scent in this context must be approached with care, combining evidence-based protocols, staff training, and a nuanced understanding of patient needs, cultural sensitivities, and room dynamics. Aromatherapy is not a substitute for clinical care but functions as a complementary modality that enhances the overall hospice environment.

Lavender is the most extensively researched essential oil in this context. Studies have consistently shown that lavender has anxiolytic properties, lowering cortisol levels, reducing heart rate, and improving subjective feelings of calm.[3] In hospice settings, the strategic diffusion of lavender during vigil hours can calm both patients and families, providing a subtle sensory cue that encourages presence, reflection, and emotional attunement. Families often remark that the first whiff of lavender creates a perceptible shift in the room's atmosphere, signaling a transition into sacred time.

Citrus-based scents such as orange, lemon, and bergamot are utilized in situations requiring alertness or gentle stimulation. For patients who may be drowsy or disengaged due to medication or illness, a faint citrus aroma can provide orientation and cognitive activation. These scents are used judiciously, never in overpowering concentrations, to ensure that the room remains tranquil while subtly guiding patient mood and engagement. Citrus aromas are particularly effective in morning or early afternoon hours, aligning scent with the patient's natural circadian rhythms.

Rosemary, peppermint, and basil are also incorporated for cognitive clarity and emotional support. In patients experiencing confusion or delirium, a light infusion of rosemary can enhance alertness and recognition of their surroundings. Careful consideration of scent intensity, ventilation, and patient sensitivity is crucial. The goal is not to impose an artificial energy but, rather, to gently support orientation and presence, reinforcing both cognitive and emotional stability.

Staff training is fundamental for effective and safe aromatherapy. Hospice professionals learn how to dilute essential oils, choose appropriate diffusion methods, and monitor patient reactions. Overconcentration can provoke nausea, respiratory irritation, or headaches. Nurses and aides are taught to observe subtle cues, such as facial expressions, body tension, and breathing patterns, to gauge whether a scent is soothing or intrusive.[4] Staff protocols also emphasize cultural and individual preferences, ensuring that aromatherapy is a supportive element rather than a prescriptive intervention.

The method of scent delivery varies depending on room size, ventilation, and patient sensitivity. Passive methods such as infused cotton pads, lightly scented linens, or sachets on memory surfaces provide gentle, localized aromatherapy. Active methods, including ultrasonic diffusers or essential oil warmers, allow for subtle diffusion over longer periods. Staff must calibrate timing, concentration, and placement, integrating scent delivery seamlessly into the existing room environment without interfering with acoustic, lighting, or tactile interventions.

A narrative illustrates the profound effect of aromatherapy in hospice care. A night-shift nurse noticed a patient exhibiting terminal restlessness: pacing the bed, vocalizing anxiously, and displaying tremors of fear. The nurse introduced a lightly diffused lavender aroma while sitting nearby, offering a gentle handhold and soft conversation. Within minutes, the patient's agitation subsided, breathing slowed, and a brief period of eye contact and connection occurred. The scent served as both a cue for calm and a tangible reassurance of presence, demonstrating how aromatherapy supports ritualized caregiving.

Multisensory integration amplifies the effectiveness of aromatherapy. Light, sound, and tactile interventions can be orchestrated alongside scent to create a cohesive emotional environment. For example, dimming bedside lights, playing soft nature sounds, and diffusing lavender together create a layered sensory experience that supports patient tranquility and family reflection. This holistic orchestration requires careful timing and sensitivity, ensuring that each modality complements the others rather than competing or overwhelming the senses.

Temporal design of aromatherapy is essential. Introducing scents only during vigil hours or during specific rituals preserves their emotional potency. Continuous or indiscriminate scent diffusion can desensitize patients, dulling the intended calming effect. By aligning aroma with the rhythm of care—morning orientation, afternoon reflection, and evening vigil—the hospice team reinforces temporal awareness and emotional continuity for both patients and families.

Cultural considerations are vital in aromatherapy design. Certain scents carry religious or spiritual significance, such as frankincense in Catholic and Orthodox traditions, sandalwood in Hindu or Buddhist practices, and sweetgrass in Indigenous rituals. Hospice staff must ensure that aromatherapy accommodates these practices, respecting ritual integrity while maintaining an inclusive environment. Integrating culturally meaningful scents enhances both emotional and spiritual resonance for families and patients.

Patient preference guides the selection of scents whenever possible. Families are encouraged to bring items from home, such as scented towels, favorite perfumes, or herbal infusions. These personal scents evoke memories and life narratives, fostering identity continuity and emotional presence. Staff often observe that familiar scents trigger recognition, emotional recall, and even verbal engagement, highlighting the power of olfactory memory in end-of-life care.

Environmental considerations include room airflow, surface absorption, and material interactions. Natural materials such as wood, wool, or cotton subtly retain aroma, extending its presence without the need for continuous diffusion. Conversely, synthetic materials may repel or neutralize scent, necessitating adjustments in delivery or concentration. Thoughtful material selection ensures that aromatherapy remains effective and harmonious with the room's overall sensory design.

Safety protocols extend to patients with respiratory vulnerabilities. Essential oils must be diluted appropriately, and ventilation should prevent accumulation of concentrated vapors. Hospice teams monitor for coughing, wheezing, or other adverse reactions, adjusting interventions as needed. By adhering to evidence-based protocols, staff ensure that aromatherapy remains a positive, nonintrusive intervention for all occupants.

Integration with other rituals reinforces the emotional significance of scent. For example, diffusing a calming aroma during hair brushing, gentle massage, or storytelling strengthens both sensory and relational cues. Families often report that these multisensory rituals create moments of deep presence, enabling both patient and loved ones to inhabit the hospice space fully.

Staff reflection is an important component of aromatherapy practice. Nurses and aides note that scent not only calms patients but also shapes their own experience of caregiving. A room with carefully curated aromatherapy provides staff with cues for slowing down; focusing attention; and engaging in deliberate, ritualized actions. This reflection enhances professional resilience and presence.

Case documentation demonstrates measurable benefits. In studies comparing standard hospice rooms to aromatherapy-integrated rooms, patients experienced lower agitation scores, reduced restlessness, and improved family satisfaction during vigil periods. Although aromatherapy is not a panacea, these findings reinforce its value as a subtle but effective component of emotional design.[5]

Aromatherapy also functions as a bridge between patient and visitor. Family members entering the room immediately sense the environment's emotional tone. The scent cues signal calm, safety, and care, allowing relatives to adjust their behavior and presence accordingly. This subtle influence strengthens communal emotional regulation, fostering a shared experience of presence and reflection.

Subtlety remains paramount. Hospice aromatherapy avoids strong, overpowering fragrances that dominate the sensory environment. The goal is to support, not overwhelm; to enhance, not replace. Light, carefully chosen scents maintain the room's quiet dignity while providing meaningful emotional and physiological support.

Diffusion methods may also be adapted to the spatial layout. Larger rooms or rooms with high ceilings require different diffusion strategies than compact spaces. Portable diffusers, passive sachets, or natural infusion through textiles can be combined to ensure even distribution without creating pockets of concentrated aroma.

Aromatherapy extends beyond patient-centered interventions. Staff may use scent in breakrooms, debrief areas, or quiet lounges to reinforce their own calm and resilience. The indirect benefits include heightened attentiveness, emotional regulation, and improved interactions with families and patients.

Ultimately, aromatherapy represents an intersection of science, art, and ritual. When integrated thoughtfully with architecture, sound, light, and tactile experiences, it contributes to a hospice environment that supports presence, dignity, and emotional continuity. Scent becomes both a therapeutic tool and a ritual anchor, embedding care, memory, and love into the very atmosphere of the hospice room.

Scent has been inseparable from human ritual for millennia, acting as both a spiritual conduit and a marker of sacred time. In hospice care, the intentional integration of culturally significant aromas—incense, herbs, flowers, and candles—supports ritualized presence and provides families with the tools to honor their beliefs while remaining in a safe, controlled environment. Each scent carries symbolic meaning: frankincense for purification and divine presence in Catholic and Orthodox Christian traditions, sandalwood and jasmine in Hindu or Buddhist rites, and sweetgrass and cedar in Indigenous ceremonies.[6] Recognizing these diverse practices requires not only knowledge of their spiritual significance but also careful adaptation to the hospice context.

When families request traditional incense, the hospice environment must accommodate this while ensuring patient safety. Many modern facilities adopt flame-free alternatives, such as LED candles or electrically heated scent diffusers that release ritual aromas without fire risk. These solutions preserve the intended symbolic function of the ritual while maintaining compliance with hospital fire codes and ventilation standards. Ventilation is crucial: Incense smoke or herb burning must not trigger alarms or overwhelm neighboring rooms.

The design of temporary ritual spaces within the room enables families to carry out scent-based traditions without disrupting other activities. Small altar tables, trays, or designated shelf surfaces allow placement of ritual objects, flowers, or incense holders. These spaces are configured to avoid crowding the patient's bedside and to maintain unobstructed staff movement, ensuring care delivery remains seamless while providing a locus for spiritual practice.

Narrative accounts illustrate the profound emotional impact of these practices. One family, observing the final days of a matriarch, set up a small altar by the window, laying down fresh flowers and using a small heated incense tray to diffuse sandalwood. The scent's gentle presence marked each step of their blessing ritual: the lighting of the incense, the whispered prayers, and the touching of sacred objects. Family members described feeling a rhythmic connection to the patient's life story, as if scent itself choreographed the ritual and aligned everyone's emotional attention.

Staff observation confirms that culturally mediated scent rituals are not solely for family benefit. Patients, even those nonverbal or semiconscious, often show physical responses: relaxed posture, slowed breathing, and fleeting expressions of recognition. These responses suggest that scent serves as a bridge between memory, spiritual belief, and immediate sensory experience, enhancing presence for both patient and family.[7]

Families sometimes bring homemade or regionally significant items, such as dried herbs, native flowers, or sacred oils. The hospice team carefully evaluates these items for safety—flammability, allergens, and contamination—while honoring their cultural value. Incorporating family-provided ritual scents reinforces continuity with the patient's home environment, reducing the sense of institutional estrangement and supporting emotional comfort.

Cultural sensitivity extends to the timing and rhythm of scent-based rituals. Certain traditions prescribe specific moments of the day for blessings or prayer, aligning scent diffusion with these temporal patterns. For example, morning incense may symbolize renewal, whereas evening diffusion may represent the transition from life to rest. Hospice staff coordinate with families to ensure these temporal preferences are honored without disturbing clinical workflows or neighboring patients.

Designing the room for scent rituals includes careful consideration of airflow and material surfaces. Aromas disperse differently depending on ceiling height, window placement, and furnishings. Soft textiles such as curtains and upholstery absorb and hold scent, creating lingering traces, whereas hard surfaces such as tile or glass reflect or dilute aromas. Understanding these dynamics allows staff to position ritual items optimally, creating an intentional and meaningful olfactory environment.

Safety protocols are paramount. Open flames are replaced with flameless alternatives whenever possible. When traditional candles or charcoal-based incense are used, they are closely monitored, placed in stable holders, and positioned away from flammable materials. Staff training emphasizes vigilance, cultural competence, and subtle guidance, ensuring rituals proceed safely without undermining their spiritual significance.

Some cultural scent practices involve layering multiple aromas simultaneously: flowers, herbs, and essential oils. This layering enhances the multisensory experience, producing complex olfactory signals that convey care, intention, and presence. Hospice teams guide families in creating balanced combinations that remain gentle, emotionally evocative, and nonintrusive for other room occupants.

The interplay between scent and light further amplifies ritual meaning. Flickering candles, real or simulated, complement the aroma, reinforcing a sense of sacred time. Shadows cast by ritual objects interact with soft, warm room illumination, creating an immersive environment that communicates reverence and tranquility without verbal direction.

Scent also functions as a mnemonic anchor, connecting ritual moments to memory and identity. Families often report that a particular aroma becomes inseparable from their recollection of the final days, preserving the emotional texture of their experience. Lavender diffused during a Hindu prayer, or frankincense during a Catholic blessing, can evoke vivid recollections years later, transforming the olfactory environment into a repository of memory.

Acoustic considerations intersect with scent rituals. Whispered prayers, chanting, or ritual singing combined with aromatic cues create a layered, multisensory ritual environment. These combinations enhance attention, deepen presence, and support shared experience. Staff may position furniture and ritual objects to optimize both sound projection and scent diffusion, ensuring the ceremony feels cohesive rather than fragmented.

Patients with cognitive impairment respond uniquely to scent. Even without conscious recognition, culturally significant aromas may trigger physiological or emotional responses, calming agitation or reinforcing a sense of belonging. Hospice staff note that patients sometimes turn toward the aroma source, close their eyes in reflective engagement, or exhibit subtle movements indicative of comfort. These observations underscore the nonverbal power of scent as a facilitator of emotional presence.

Family education is critical. Staff guide relatives in safe and effective use of scent, including dosage, timing, and placement. They provide culturally informed alternatives when traditional items cannot be safely used, such as electric incense holders or herbal infusions. Families gain confidence in performing rituals, knowing that both patient safety and spiritual integrity are maintained.

Scent rituals often mark transitions within the hospice experience. The onset of vigil hours, the completion of a blessing, or the moment of final repose may be accompanied by intentional diffusion or extinguishing of ritual scents. These olfactory cues act as signals, guiding attention and facilitating collective recognition of important temporal and emotional milestones.

Integration with other sensory modalities enhances ritual depth. Tactile interactions with ritual objects, gentle music, and visual cues such as light or color coordinate with olfactory signals, producing an enveloping environment conducive to reflection, connection, and closure. This orchestration requires careful staff facilitation to prevent sensory overload while sustaining the emotional resonance of the ritual.

Documentation of scent rituals provides continuity for incoming staff. Notes regarding preferred aromas, timing, and family practices allow caregivers to maintain consistency across shifts, preserving ritual integrity and patient comfort. Such attention to detail signals respect for the family's cultural values and supports the therapeutic alliance between staff and loved ones.

Beyond the immediate room, scent practices influence the emotional tone of communal hospice spaces. Corridors, shared lounges, and entryways may carry subtle residual aromas from ritualized rooms, creating an overarching atmosphere of calm, dignity, and spiritual attentiveness.

Ultimately, cultural and spiritual scent rituals transform the hospice room from a clinical setting into a sacred, multisensory space. By integrating aroma thoughtfully with architecture, light, sound, and tactile elements, hospice design honors the diverse beliefs of patients and families, supports emotional and spiritual well-being, and preserves the continuity of life's most significant moments.

Hospice rooms operate under strict hygiene and infection control protocols. The need for cleanliness is paramount, as patients are often immunocompromised and highly susceptible to pathogens. Yet, the pursuit of sterility can inadvertently strip the environment of warmth, intimacy, and sensory comfort. A room that smells sharply of antiseptic wipes, disinfectant sprays, or hospital-grade cleaners can evoke anxiety and distance, reminding patients and families of the clinical setting rather than fostering emotional presence. Balancing hygiene with olfactory warmth is therefore a critical design and operational challenge in the creation of compassionate hospice spaces.

The integration of scent into hospice care must respect infection control while simultaneously providing emotional and sensory support. Staff are trained to select natural, subtle fragrances that are non-irritating, non-allergenic, and easily removable if necessary. Essential oils, herbal infusions, and scent diffusers are deployed strategically, maintaining a delicate balance between olfactory enrichment and sanitary compliance. Diffusers are cleaned regularly, and replacement protocols ensure that residues do not accumulate and interfere with hygienic standards.

A central principle is that scent should never compete with hygiene but complement it. For example, clinical odors from cleaning agents or bodily functions can be softened or masked without introducing overpowering fragrances. Mild lavender, chamomile, or citrus blends can reduce clinical sterility and evoke domestic familiarity, helping patients feel emotionally "at home" even in a medicalized environment. The goal is not to cover odors artificially but to create a gentle olfactory background that supports comfort and presence.

Spatial considerations also influence scent deployment. Diffusers are placed away from high-traffic areas, ventilation intakes, or the bedside to avoid overconcentration. Some hospice units integrate ceiling-mounted systems or concealed wall diffusers, allowing fragrances to circulate subtly. These systems are programmable, enabling staff to adjust intensity or timing based on patient sensitivity, family preference, or room occupancy. The design ensures that scent enhances the emotional environment without interfering with clinical care.

Narrative accounts reveal the impact of scent on family perception of the hospice environment. One family recounted that subtle herbal aromas brought the room closer to the patient's home, transforming the perception from a "sterile hospital ward" into a space of warmth and memory. These olfactory cues were instrumental in helping relatives relax, focus on presence, and participate meaningfully in ritual activities.

The careful choice of scent also reduces sensory overload. Strong perfumes, incense, or overly synthetic fragrances can provoke headaches, nausea, or discomfort, particularly among fragile patients. Staff training emphasizes moderation, cultural sensitivity, and observation of patient reactions, allowing scent deployment to be tailored individually. Diffusers are often paired with other sensory interventions, such as soft lighting, comfortable textiles, and familiar objects, reinforcing the room's emotional coherence.

Infection control policies require that items introducing scent, such as essential oil diffusers or herbal trays, are regularly sanitized or replaced. Containers holding liquids or powders must be leak-proof and cleaned to prevent microbial growth. These procedures ensure that the introduction of sensory warmth does not compromise safety, and they reinforce family confidence in the care environment.

The juxtaposition of hygiene and olfactory warmth also informs textile and material choices. Bedding, curtains, and upholstery are selected for both cleanability and scent retention. Natural fibers such as cotton, linen, or wool can absorb and diffuse gentle aromas, creating lingering olfactory impressions, whereas synthetic or heavily treated fabrics may repel scent or harbor chemicals that interfere with sensory cues. Furniture, walls, and flooring surfaces are similarly chosen to support hygiene while allowing fragrance to remain perceptible without contamination.

Temporal management of scent is equally important. During clinical procedures, scent diffusion may be temporarily paused to avoid interference with procedural odor detection or sterilization processes. After procedures, scent can be reintroduced gradually, marking a transition back to vigil hours or restful periods. This subtle temporal orchestration strengthens the room's emotional rhythm, signaling changes in care phases without verbal instruction.

Case studies illustrate practical applications. In one hospice unit, staff observed that patients with terminal restlessness calmed noticeably when mild lavender diffusers were activated during the evening hours. The aroma was carefully adjusted to avoid overpowering the room, and devices were cleaned daily to maintain hygiene. Families reported that the combination of subtle scent, soft lighting, and familiar blankets created a sense of continuity with the patient's home environment, reducing stress for both patient and visitors.

The balance between hygiene and scent also intersects with staff workflow. Nurses and aides are trained to position diffusers in accessible yet safe locations, allowing adjustments without compromising bed access or emergency protocols. Scent systems are often coordinated with cleaning routines to prevent conflicts between fragrance and disinfectant use, ensuring a seamless operational rhythm.

Scent can serve as an emotional bridge for families during moments of grief. When diffusers are activated during final conversations or vigils, the familiar aroma reinforces memory formation and presence. Families report that the room, imbued with subtle olfactory cues, feels "alive" with the patient's essence, providing comfort and continuity even after death.

Cultural sensitivity remains paramount. Certain families may find specific aromas inappropriate or incongruent with their traditions. Staff collaborate with relatives to select alternatives that honor belief systems while preserving hygiene standards. Options include flameless candles, herbal sachets, or aromatherapy pads, all carefully monitored for cleanliness and safety.

The integration of scent with other sensory modalities enhances therapeutic effect. Coordinated use with soundscapes, lighting, and tactile objects creates a multisensory environment that fosters calm, presence, and ritual participation. For example, a soft fragrance combined with gentle instrumental music and a warm throw blanket produces an enveloping sense of security and home-like familiarity.

Staff observation confirms that the subtle management of scent reduces distress not only for patients but also for family members. The olfactory environment contributes to perceived room quality, impacting willingness to remain at the bedside, engage in ritual, and participate in emotional closure. Maintaining this balance is a continuous practice, requiring attentiveness and adaptation.

Operational protocols include monitoring for patient sensitivity. Some patients may have respiratory conditions or heightened olfactory perception, necessitating the temporary reduction or removal of scent. Staff document preferences and reactions, ensuring that subsequent shifts maintain consistency in both hygiene and sensory warmth.

Design strategies also support seasonal variation. Diffusers may adjust intensity or type of aroma based on ambient temperature, humidity, or seasonal plant availability, enhancing the perception of a living, responsive environment. This dynamic approach reinforces the room's role as a companion through changing times and states of being.

Ultimately, balancing hygiene with sensory warmth transforms hospice rooms from sterile clinical spaces into environments that nurture emotional presence, support ritual, and sustain dignity. This equilibrium requires architectural foresight, staff training, cultural sensitivity, and careful operational management. When achieved, it enhances patient comfort, facilitates family engagement, and preserves the subtle yet powerful role of scent in the architecture of care.

In hospice care, scent can serve as a subtle but profoundly effective guide for the emotional rhythms of a room. In addition to comfort or memory recall, scent can signal transitions in care, mark the start of vigil hours, or gently cue the evening reflection period. These olfactory cues operate without verbal instruction, creating a quiet, shared understanding between staff, patients, and families. They are a nonverbal language of presence, anticipation, and ritual, underscoring the temporal and emotional flow of the day.

Staff often describe scent as a bridge between intention and experience. When a diffuser releases a calming lavender or chamomile aroma at the start of vigil hours, families intuitively understand that this is a period for quiet observation, reflection, or prayer. The smell becomes part of the rhythm, guiding the collective attention of everyone in the room toward presence and stillness. It signals that clinical routines are secondary to human connection in these moments.

The orchestration of scent as an emotional guide is inherently multisensory. It aligns with light modulation, soft soundscapes, and tactile cues such as the placement of a warm blanket or the soft hum of an essential oil diffuser. When synchronized, these sensory layers produce a holistic experience in which patients feel comforted, families feel invited into ritual, and staff can perform care with emotional intentionality.

Narratives from family members reveal the emotional potency of scent cues. One daughter recounted that the gradual release of a subtle lavender aroma during evening vigil hours "softened the room" and allowed her to shift from anxiety to a reflective presence. She described noticing a mental and emotional pathway form in the room, a rhythm she could follow, where attention moved naturally from observing breath patterns to sharing memories without needing verbal guidance.

Staff reflections emphasize the careful calibration required to achieve this effect. Patients vary widely in olfactory sensitivity, respiratory tolerance, and cultural preference. For some, a faint scent is sufficient; for others, even a mild aroma may be overwhelming. Nurses and aides are trained to observe patient response, adjust intensity, and rotate scents according to both individual needs and family expectations. This requires ongoing communication, documentation, and sensitivity to context.

Diffuser placement is as critical as scent selection. Strategically embedding scent delivery into architectural elements—such as concealed wall diffusers, ceiling panels, or bedside furniture—allows aroma to disperse naturally throughout the room. This ensures that scent is part of the spatial experience rather than an external or intrusive element, creating a seamless emotional architecture.

The timing of scent release reinforces the room's temporal structure. For example, a brief pulse of a soothing aroma at the start of vigil signals the shift from daytime activity to evening reflection. A different scent might accompany routine nursing care, subtly cueing families that certain interactions are necessary but not central to presence. These transitions are invisible yet profoundly felt, creating a subconscious rhythm that supports emotional stability.

Case studies highlight the efficacy of scent as an emotional guide. In one hospice unit, families reported that the consistent use of mild chamomile during evening reflection helped reduce anticipatory anxiety before a patient's final hours. The fragrance, combined with soft lighting and gentle instrumental music, produced a cohesive environment that facilitated presence, storytelling, and ritual engagement.

Olfactory cues can also guide staff behavior. When diffusers release a particular aroma, nurses recognize that they are entering a period that prioritizes vigil and reflection over procedural efficiency. This helps prevent inadvertent disruption of sacred time, ensuring that staff movements are measured, quiet, and aligned with the emotional tone of the room. In this sense, scent acts as both a patient-centered and staff-centered guide.

Families often internalize scent as a mnemonic device. After leaving the hospice, returning to the same fragrance—lavender, sandalwood, or citrus—can evoke recollection of vigil hours, conversations, and shared rituals. Scent becomes part of the memory-keeping architecture, allowing emotional presence to extend beyond the physical room. This reinforces the temporal continuity of care and the enduring significance of small rituals.

The psychological mechanisms behind scent as an emotional guide are well-documented. Olfactory signals connect directly to the limbic system, influencing mood, memory, and stress responses. Unlike other senses, smell bypasses the rational cortex, allowing subconscious emotional regulation and creating immediate physiological effects such as reduced heart rate, lower cortisol levels, and increased relaxation. This physiological grounding enhances both patient comfort and family engagement.

Cultural sensitivity shapes scent selection and timing. Different traditions associate particular fragrances with mourning, blessing, or spiritual presence. Staff collaborate with families to select appropriate aromas, ensuring that scent reinforces ritual rather than contradicting cultural norms. For example, incense may be used in flame-free forms to honor religious traditions without violating safety or hygiene protocols.

Integration with other architectural and design elements strengthens the impact of scent. Soft textiles, tactile objects, and warm lighting amplify olfactory cues, creating a multisensory scaffold for ritual and reflection. A familiar blanket carrying a faint scent from home can be layered with diffuser-based aromas to extend memory and emotional continuity.

Scent also marks physical transitions in the room. The start of an evening vigil, the preparation for a final conversation, or the shift from care activities to contemplative reflection can each be subtly signaled with specific aromas. Families quickly learn these cues, which reduce the need for verbal explanation and allow presence to emerge organically.

The use of scent requires careful consideration of duration. Continuous fragrance can become overwhelming, losing its emotional subtlety. Short, intentional pulses of aroma are more effective, creating ephemeral yet meaningful cues that align with the temporal flow of care.

Diffusers may be synchronized with natural elements. For example, a soft floral aroma might accompany the rising sun in morning reflection periods, whereas evening vigils use calming herbal scents. This creates a poetic echo of natural cycles, aligning patient experience with the rhythms of day and night.

Staff note that scent can also mitigate anticipatory grief and anxiety in families. When the room carries a familiar, soothing aroma, relatives are less distracted by clinical odors or the sterile ambiance of a hospital-adjacent environment. This allows for deeper engagement with the patient, more meaningful participation in ritual, and greater emotional resilience.

Design implications extend beyond individual rooms. Hallways, lounges, and family waiting areas may carry subtle scent cues that extend the hospice's emotional architecture throughout the unit. These cues can provide continuity, helping families transition from shared spaces to private vigil rooms while maintaining emotional grounding.

Safety remains a central concern. All scent interventions must comply with infection control, respiratory safety, and allergy protocols. Staff are trained to monitor patient response, adjust delivery, and remove scent sources if adverse reactions occur. The emotional benefits of olfactory guidance must always be weighed against physiological risk.

Ultimately, scent as an emotional guide exemplifies how architecture, ritual, and care converge in hospice environments. When thoughtfully integrated, scent cues orchestrate transitions, support multisensory engagement, and provide families and staff with a shared emotional framework. The hospice room becomes not only a space for presence but also a living, breathing participant in the rhythms of care.

9
Invisible Tools for Comfort

Hospice environments are often imagined as spaces free from technological intrusion, emphasizing warmth, ritual, and human presence. Yet, when thoughtfully integrated, subtle technology can enhance comfort and emotional experience without diminishing dignity. Smart environment systems—including automated lighting, climate control, and shading—allow the room itself to respond to the needs of patients, families, and staff, creating a more humane and seamless experience.

Automated lighting systems are central to these smart environments. Rather than requiring a family member or staff member to adjust switches repeatedly, lights can respond to circadian rhythms, gradually dimming as evening vigil hours approach and brightening gently in the morning to signal reflection or care routines.[1] The room becomes a silent participant, providing guidance through intuitive illumination.

For patients, these automated systems reduce the sensory burden of decision-making.[2] Those nearing the end of life often have limited energy or mobility. By allowing the environment to respond predictably, technology conserves cognitive and physical energy, letting the patient focus on presence rather than the mechanics of controlling light, temperature, or blinds. Families immediately perceive this as relief, creating an atmosphere of trust in the room's capacity for care.

Climate control is another critical feature. Intelligent thermostats can maintain warmth without sudden drafts, automatically adjusting to outside weather or patient activity.[3] For patients sensitive to temperature fluctuations, the system stabilizes comfort without intrusive manual intervention. Families often describe the emotional impact of entering a room in which temperature feels "just right," noting that it conveys a subtle but profound attentiveness to the patient's needs.

Shading and window automation offer a nuanced form of control over natural light. Smart shades can tilt or lift gradually to prevent glare on the patient while maintaining visual access to the outdoors. For example, a patient may benefit from viewing the morning sun without the discomfort of direct rays. The room's design is thus actively participating in both comfort and emotional well-being.

A key narrative emerges when technology subtly reduces cognitive load for families. One family recounted that during a night vigil, automated dimming and temperature adjustment allowed them to focus entirely on shared presence and ritual. They did not need to think about turning off lights, adjusting the thermostat, or opening blinds—they could simply be present. This invisibility of technology enhances emotional flow rather than distracting from it.

Smart environment systems also enhance staff efficiency. When lighting, sound, and climate are automated, nurses and aides can anticipate changes without manual intervention, leaving their attention free for intimate care tasks. This supports the choreography of movement and ritual within the room, reducing both physical strain and emotional stress.

Safety protocols are another benefit. Automated systems can detect open windows in cold weather, sudden temperature drops, or malfunctioning heating, ventilation, and air-conditioning (HVAC) systems, alerting staff to intervene before the patient experiences discomfort. These systems function quietly in the background, maintaining dignity while ensuring environmental safety.

Technology allows nuanced temporal signaling. For example, lighting changes, combined with slight shifts in climate or airflow, can signal the start of vigil hours without verbal instruction.[4] Families intuitively recognize these cues, reinforcing continuity of care and ritualized behavior. This multisensory orchestration is a hallmark of next-generation hospice design.

In addition to function, smart systems contribute to spatial and emotional coherence. By maintaining consistent lighting levels, subtle climate adjustments, and adaptive shading, these technologies prevent visual or tactile disruption that could create anxiety. The patient perceives a stable environment, enhancing feelings of safety and predictability, which are essential in end-of-life care.[5]

Narratives of patient experience illustrate the emotional resonance. One hospice patient commented that the automated lighting and soft airflow "felt like the room was breathing with me." Such reports highlight the importance of designing technology that is not only functional but also emotionally intelligent, capable of supporting the psychological needs of those in transition.

Integration with other sensory modalities strengthens the effect. For instance, light, sound, and scent can be coordinated through smart systems, producing a gentle orchestration of mood and ritual. A diffuser releasing calming aroma synchronized with dimming lights signals the start of evening vigil. This creates a multisensory rhythm, reinforcing ritual and emotional presence.

Ethical design underpins smart environments. Technology must never replace human presence or interaction. Instead, it serves as an invisible scaffold, supporting human care rather than supplanting it. Staff training emphasizes that automation is a complement to attentive caregiving, not a substitute for relational engagement.

The architecture itself can integrate these systems invisibly. Ceiling panels, wall niches, or built-in furniture can house sensors, diffusers, and automated controls. The goal is for technology to dissolve into the space, reinforcing calm and continuity rather than introducing a clinical or artificial aesthetic.

Patient-centered design requires customization. Systems should allow staff and families to override automation when needed, tailoring light, temperature, and shading to specific preferences. This flexibility supports individual needs while maintaining the emotional and ritual continuity of the room.

Longitudinal observation demonstrates the cumulative impact. Families returning to the same hospice space over multiple days notice consistent environmental behavior, which fosters a sense of security and trust. Repeated exposure to stable, responsive conditions strengthens the perception of the room as a compassionate, attentive presence.

Integration of smart systems must account for cultural and spiritual variation. For example, certain religious rituals may require specific light levels, timing, or shading conditions. Advanced systems can be programmed to honor these needs without staff intervention, supporting inclusivity and respectful care.

Technology also supports the reduction of disruptive environmental elements. Alarms, sudden HVAC changes, or bright task lights can be muted or gradually modulated, ensuring that human presence and ritual remain central. Subtlety is critical: Patients and families should not perceive technology as intrusive or artificial.

Staff narratives underscore the emotional relief provided by invisible technology. One nurse reported that smart climate and lighting adjustments allowed her to focus entirely on a patient's final moments, observing breath and subtle expressions rather than worrying about environmental controls. This reduces cognitive load and enhances the quality of bedside presence.

Finally, smart environment systems exemplify how architecture, ritual, and technology can harmonize in hospice care. When thoughtfully designed, automation respects human dignity, reinforces emotional and ritual continuity, and enhances both patient and family experience. The room itself becomes an active participant in care, unobtrusively guiding attention, supporting presence, and preserving the sacredness of end-of-life moments.

Discreet patient monitoring in hospice environments represents a careful balance between safety, dignity, and emotional tranquility. Unlike traditional hospital monitoring, which can be invasive and disruptive, contemporary systems are designed to operate silently in the background. Sensors and monitors track vital signs, movement, and potential hazards without the overt presence of devices, alarms, or intrusive equipment.

The use of noncontact sensors has revolutionized end-of-life care.[6] Bed-based systems detect subtle changes in heart rate, respiration, and movement patterns, alerting staff only when thresholds indicate potential distress. Families and patients often report feeling less observed, reducing anxiety and creating a sense of freedom within the room. The patient's environment becomes more like a home than a clinical ward.

Vital sign monitoring is critical for managing discomfort or sudden medical complications. Advanced sensors detect irregular breathing patterns or heart rate fluctuations, immediately notifying staff. Yet, unlike traditional monitoring, there are no flashing screens or audible beeps unless intervention is required. This preserves the emotional calm of the room, supporting the rituals and quiet attention essential to hospice care.

Fall-prevention technology is another key element. Pressure-sensitive floor mats or motion sensors can alert staff when a patient attempts to leave the bed without assistance. The alerts are routed discreetly, often to wearable devices or silent pagers, minimizing disruption for both patient and family.[7] These systems prevent accidents without introducing the fear or hyper-vigilance often associated with constant observation.

Narratives from families reveal the subtle impact of this technology. One family recounted that their loved one was able to sleep deeply, undisturbed by monitoring equipment, yet the family and staff were confident that the patient would be attended to immediately if needed. This dual perception—safety without intrusion—is foundational to discreet monitoring.

Ethical considerations are paramount. Patients and families must consent to monitoring and understand its function. Transparency builds trust: Explaining that sensors work silently, only alerting staff in critical situations, allows families to engage fully with the patient without fear of violating privacy. Autonomy and dignity are preserved when patients understand that the room's technology supports them rather than surveilling them.

Discreet monitoring also supports staff workflow. Nurses can monitor multiple rooms with minimal physical disruption, allowing them to prioritize time for direct caregiving, ritual support, and emotional presence. This integration enhances professional efficiency without sacrificing the human-centered focus central to hospice philosophy.

Integration with the broader smart environment enhances functionality. Vital sign alerts can trigger small, automated adjustments—subtle lighting changes, airflow modulation, or sound cues—to respond to discomfort nonintrusively. For example, a slight increase in airflow combined with dimmed lights may indicate a comfortable adjustment when respiratory patterns change, often before a patient or family member even notices.

The technology is particularly beneficial for patients experiencing delirium, terminal restlessness, or cognitive impairment. By reducing intrusive interventions and maintaining environmental predictability, monitoring devices support mental and emotional stability while ensuring rapid response to physical needs. Families often report that this creates a sense of security and calm that directly affects their own ability to be present.

Discreet monitoring also complements other sensory interventions. When combined with smart lighting, soundscapes, or scent diffusion, sensors provide real-time feedback to ensure comfort and maintain ritual continuity. A shift in vital signs might prompt a subtle adjustment in the room's environment, reinforcing care without verbal interruption.

Staff training is crucial for maximizing the benefits of discreet monitoring. Clinicians must interpret sensor data appropriately, respond quickly when required, and avoid overreliance on technology. The goal is always to preserve the human touch, ensuring that interventions remain compassionate and informed by emotional context as well as physiological data.

The design of sensor systems emphasizes invisibility. Devices are integrated into bed frames, ceiling panels, or furniture. This preserves spatial coherence and avoids triggering clinical associations that can provoke anxiety or distress. Patients and families often note that technology "disappears" into the room, allowing the space to retain its warmth, ritual function, and sense of home.

Privacy extends beyond the room itself. Data transmission is encrypted and secured, accessible only to authorized staff. Families are reassured that monitoring is a protective measure, not an invasive surveillance system, supporting both ethical responsibility and emotional trust.

One family described a night vigil in which the patient moved slightly, triggering a silent alert. Staff arrived within moments, without the disruption of alarms or rushing equipment. The patient continued sleeping peacefully, the family remained present, and the room maintained its calm. This narrative illustrates the intersection of safety, dignity, and emotional continuity.

Patient-centered customization is also vital. Families and patients can adjust sensitivity thresholds or notification preferences in collaboration with staff, ensuring that monitoring aligns with individual comfort and care goals. For example, a patient with terminal agitation may require more frequent observation, whereas another may benefit from a more passive monitoring mode.

Nonintrusive monitoring supports bereavement continuity as well. Families often feel reassured that even after they have temporarily left the room, their loved one remains safe. This contributes to reduced anxiety and allows family members to rest, meditate, or engage in other rituals without constant physical presence.

The combination of environmental monitoring and human-centered automation enables predictive care. By observing patterns over time, staff can anticipate needs, adjusting comfort measures proactively rather than reactively.[8] This predictive capacity strengthens the sense of attentiveness that families experience in the room.

Monitoring technology also facilitates interdisciplinary communication. Alerts and logs can be shared with physicians, nurses, and chaplains in a coordinated manner, ensuring that interventions—whether clinical, emotional, or spiritual—are harmonized. Families notice the seamless integration of staff attention and care coordination, which reinforces trust and emotional security.

The presence of discreet monitoring also supports ethical end-of-life decision-making. By providing continuous data without intruding on presence, families and clinicians are empowered to make informed choices regarding comfort interventions, medication adjustments, or ritual timing with confidence.

Finally, discreet patient monitoring exemplifies the subtle interplay of technology, architecture, and ritual in hospice spaces. By safeguarding physical well-being, preserving emotional integrity, and allowing space for human presence, these systems embody the ethos of a next-generation hospice room: supportive, unobtrusive, and profoundly humane.

Virtual presence technologies have emerged as a critical tool in modern hospice care, allowing families and loved ones to participate in the end-of-life experience even when physical attendance is impossible. Audio and video systems can be seamlessly integrated into patient rooms, enabling participation without disrupting the sacred calm of the space. These systems extend the notion of presence beyond physical boundaries, creating a new layer of ritual and connection.

The emotional significance of virtual presence cannot be overstated. Families separated by distance, illness, or travel restrictions can now witness vigil hours, prayers, or personal reflections without feeling excluded.[9] Patients often experience comfort knowing their loved ones are visually or audibly present, reinforcing a sense of continuity and identity in their final days.

A core principle in designing virtual presence systems is subtlety. Devices are carefully positioned to avoid drawing attention, cluttering the room, or creating a clinical atmosphere. Cameras are integrated into furniture or mounted discreetly, while microphones capture clear sound without requiring intrusive placement near the patient. The architecture and interior design continue to prioritize tranquility and visual simplicity.

One patient's family recounted using a tablet during a vigil to connect a grandchild who lived far away. The device was placed on a small table in the reflection zone, allowing the grandchild to speak, read stories, and even sing softly. The child's presence did not disturb the room's emotional tone; rather, it enhanced the intimacy of the moment, reinforcing the family's sense of collective witnessing.

Staff play a critical role in mediating virtual presence. Nurses and hospice aides ensure that technology operates smoothly, manage audio levels, and coordinate participation while maintaining the dignity and privacy of the patient. The presence of staff also ensures that technological mediation does not replace the human touch but instead complements it.

Virtual presence can also facilitate spiritual guidance. Chaplains, clergy, or spiritual mentors can join remotely, offering prayers, readings, or rituals in real time. Families report that these remote interventions feel as intimate as in-person attendance, provided the technology is thoughtfully implemented and sensitive to visual and auditory aesthetics.

Case studies highlight the power of these systems. In one instance, an elderly patient was comforted during their final hours by the remote presence of a distant sibling. The sibling recited poetry and shared memories, creating an emotional bridge across miles. The patient's breathing patterns slowed, and family members present noted an enhanced sense of calm, demonstrating that virtual presence can support physiological and emotional regulation simultaneously.

Audio quality is critical. High-fidelity microphones capture speech and whispered stories, while speakers or headphones are configured to maintain a gentle, enveloping sound environment. Poor audio quality or intrusive feedback can break the emotional intimacy, emphasizing the need for careful acoustic integration within the room.

Video framing is equally important. Patients should never feel "on display." Camera placement emphasizes a shared experience rather than surveillance.[10] Wide-angle lenses can capture the family circle without focusing solely on the patient, allowing virtual attendees to witness rituals, lighting changes, or symbolic gestures in context.

One narrative described a hospice room in which multiple family members joined via video simultaneously. Staff coordinated the session so that each person had a turn to speak or observe without creating a fragmented or chaotic experience. The technology became an invisible facilitator of collective presence rather than a disruptive novelty.

Privacy considerations are paramount. Virtual sessions are encrypted, access-controlled, and monitored to prevent unauthorized viewing. Families and patients are guided through consent protocols, reinforcing trust and ensuring that technology operates ethically. This framework mirrors the overarching hospice commitment to dignity and confidentiality.

Integration with other sensory elements enhances the effect of virtual presence. For example, when a loved one recites prayers remotely, the room's lighting might subtly dim, or a gentle scent diffuser could release calming aromas. The synchronization of visual, auditory, and olfactory cues reinforces ritual and presence, making virtual connection feel emotionally holistic.

Staff reflections emphasize that virtual presence should never replace in-room caregiving. Technology is a bridge, not a substitute. Nurses and aides maintain physical presence, providing touch, guidance, and reassurance. Virtual tools augment human care, extending emotional reach without diminishing personal connection.

Families often report that virtual presence allows participation in intimate rituals they could not otherwise attend—singing, storytelling, or symbolic acts such as lighting a candle. The knowledge that their presence was "felt" contributes to closure, grief processing, and a sense of fulfillment for both patient and family.

Cultural sensitivity is critical. Different traditions may have distinct expectations regarding witnessing, ritual participation, and physical proximity. Virtual presence systems must be flexible enough to accommodate various cultural and spiritual practices while preserving the room's aesthetic and emotional integrity.

One challenge noted by staff is the potential for technical distractions. Even subtle glitches can interrupt ritual flow, underscoring the importance of preprogrammed, tested setups. Redundancy in systems—backup devices, precharged batteries, and clear instructions—ensures reliability during critical moments.

Time zone differences present unique opportunities and challenges. Remote family members may join at unconventional hours. Staff mediate these situations, adjusting room lighting and environmental cues to align with both the patient's circadian comfort and the emotional needs of virtual attendees.

Emotional narratives consistently highlight the long-term impact of virtual presence. Family members describe lingering comfort in knowing they were "there" even from afar. Patients often comment on the reassurance of seeing familiar faces or hearing loved ones' voices, reinforcing a sense of continuity and identity until the final moments.

The integration of virtual presence into hospice care also prompts design implications for future rooms. Ports, cabling, and device mounts should be concealed, maintaining clean sightlines. Furniture arrangements must allow cameras to capture meaningful angles without imposing on the family's spatial rituals. In this way, technology respects both functional and emotional architecture.

In summary, virtual presence in hospice care exemplifies the careful balance between technological facilitation and human-centered design. When implemented thoughtfully, it enhances emotional presence, supports ritual continuity, and strengthens connections across distance, all while preserving dignity and the sacred calm of the hospice room. The technology is not the story itself; it is a conduit for shared witnessing, compassion, and the continuity of life and memory.

Technology in hospice care is often thought of as clinical or utilitarian, yet it has profound potential to support ritual and meaning. Audio playback systems, ambient sound controls, and integrated lighting cues can serve as unobtrusive facilitators of end-of-life rituals.[11] By aligning technical functionality with emotional and spiritual needs, these systems reinforce the continuity of care while honoring the sacred rhythms of hospice life.

One of the primary tools in supporting ritual is audio playback. Families can select prerecorded prayers, songs, storytelling sessions, or spoken poetry that carry deep personal or cultural significance. When played at appropriate volumes, these recordings transform the room into a space of memory, reflection, and reverence. The technology allows families to guide ritual without monopolizing staff attention, enabling care providers to focus on physical and emotional support.

Ambient soundscapes further enhance the ritual experience. Gentle rainfall, wind in trees, or distant waves can be synchronized with vigil hours, marking transitions without overt announcement. The interplay between natural sound cues and recorded voices creates an emotional layering that reinforces the sacredness of the moment. The room itself becomes a living participant in ritual rather than a passive backdrop.

Lighting cues are another subtle yet profound tool. Dimming sequences, color temperature adjustments, and spotlighting can correspond with ceremonial moments.[12] For instance, a bedside lamp might gradually warm as a family gathers for reflection, signaling the start of vigil hours, while soft dimming cues mark the end of active rituals. These visual signals serve as nonverbal guides for both family and staff, embedding temporal structure into the experience.

Narratives from families illustrate the emotional resonance of technology in ritual. One family utilized recordings of ancestral prayers to guide nightly vigil rhythm. As the recordings played, family members positioned themselves around the patient, taking turns reciting responses, lighting symbolic candles, and holding hands. The audio system ensured that the prayer cycle could proceed uninterrupted, even when distant relatives contributed remotely, creating a sense of communal participation.

Staff observations highlight the emotional impact of such systems. Nurses reported that when ritual sounds and lighting were used intentionally, patients often became visibly calmer. Heart rates normalized; facial tension decreased; and families expressed gratitude for a structured, meaningful experience. Technology here does not replace the human element; it amplifies it, providing a framework in which care, presence, and ritual coexist harmoniously.

Integration of technology must always be unobtrusive. Devices should not dominate sightlines or interfere with furniture placement. Speakers can be recessed into walls or hidden within cabinetry, while lighting controls are embedded into bedside panels or mobile apps. The goal is to create a seamless experience in which technology disappears into the architecture, leaving only the emotional and ritual experience in focus.

Flexibility is essential. Different families and patients have diverse preferences, cultural norms, and spiritual practices. Systems must allow customization of audio, light, and even timing sequences. A Catholic family might use hymn playback, whereas a Buddhist family prefers chanting and bell sequences. Technology should accommodate both traditions without privileging one over another, maintaining inclusivity and respect.

Narratives also demonstrate the layering of human and technological presence. A hospice nurse recalled a patient whose family used recorded lullabies sung by distant grandchildren. As the music played, the nurse facilitated a gentle hand massage and positioned a comforting blanket, synchronizing tactile, auditory, and visual cues. The combined sensory orchestration reinforced connection, dignity, and ritual continuity.

Case studies indicate that technology can support complex ceremonies. Some families integrate narrative storytelling, music therapy, and candlelight—all mediated by technology—to create multidimensional rituals. Even in small rooms, devices allow these practices without crowding or overwhelming the patient, preserving both intimacy and spatial coherence.

Training staff to use ritual-supportive technologies is crucial. Intuitive interfaces, clear protocols, and quick-access controls reduce cognitive load and prevent errors during emotionally charged moments. Staff must understand both technical operation and the symbolic meaning of cues to mediate experiences effectively.

The ethical dimension cannot be overlooked. Systems must respect patient autonomy and consent. Families and patients should guide which rituals are played, when, and for whom. Overly prescriptive or automated interventions risk undermining dignity and emotional control, emphasizing the importance of human oversight.

Cultural sensitivity extends to sound choice and volume. Loud or intrusive playback can unintentionally distress patients or families. Conversely, subtle, soft sounds convey care, presence, and reverence. The integration of volume sliders, directional speakers, and audio equalization allows for precise control that respects both patient needs and ritual integrity.

Families consistently describe enhanced emotional closure when technology supports rituals. One narrative describes the final vigil of a patient whose children lived abroad. By synchronizing recorded songs, prayer sequences, and guided storytelling, the family could "be present" collectively. The technology became a bridge for shared experience, fostering closure without compromising the sanctity of the room.

The design of the environment itself interacts with technology to support rituals. Walls, flooring, and ceiling materials affect sound quality, and furniture placement determines acoustic pathways. Integrating devices with these architectural features ensures that the ritual signals are clear, harmonious, and emotionally resonant.

Technological redundancy is important. Backup devices, precharged batteries, and cloud-based audio storage ensure that rituals are uninterrupted even during power outages or technical glitches. Families find comfort in knowing that rituals will proceed as intended, minimizing anxiety during critical moments.

Staff reflections emphasize that ritual-supportive technology fosters emotional resilience. By offloading some ritual facilitation to reliable systems, caregivers can focus on relational presence. The technology acts as a framework or scaffold, allowing nurses and aides to direct attention toward subtle human cues, bedside care, and emotional accompaniment.

Temporal structuring is enhanced through technology. Lighting dimmers and audio cues create gentle transitions between day and night, care and reflection, active monitoring and rest. This temporal orchestration provides families with a sense of rhythm, marking sacred time without verbal instruction or disruption.

Future implications suggest that hospice design can incorporate these systems at the architectural level. Built-in speakers, lighting rails, and dedicated control panels allow ritual technology to be fully integrated into the room's fabric. These interventions can support multisensory ritual without clutter or distraction, reinforcing the concept of the room as an active participant in hospice care.

Ultimately, technology in ritual support demonstrates that human-centered design can harmonize with emotional and spiritual practice. When thoughtfully implemented, it enhances continuity, dignity, and emotional connection. Families and patients experience care that is both sensitive and structured, while staff maintain the sacred calm essential to hospice environments.

Hospice care exists at the intersection of vulnerability, dignity, and deep human connection. Introducing technology into this intimate space requires careful ethical consideration. Although systems for monitoring, communication, and ritual facilitation can enhance safety and comfort, they can also inadvertently disrupt privacy, autonomy, and emotional space if implemented thoughtlessly. Ethical guidelines ensure that technology supports rather than supplants the core human-centered mission of hospice.

At the foundation of ethical technology use is consent. Patients, whenever capable, should be informed about any monitoring devices, recording systems, or automated interventions. Consent must be ongoing and revisitable, especially in cases in which cognitive status may fluctuate near the end of life. Even well-intentioned interventions can feel intrusive if the patient or family is unaware of their presence.

For patients unable to provide consent, surrogate decision-makers play a central role. Families should be fully briefed on the capabilities, limitations, and intended use of any technology. Decisions must prioritize the patient's dignity, comfort, and spiritual preferences, rather than convenience for staff or institutional efficiency. Ethical frameworks guide staff in weighing benefit against potential harm.

Privacy is paramount. Sensors for movement, vital signs, or audio monitoring must avoid constant observation beyond what is necessary for safety. Systems that capture video should be carefully restricted, encrypted, and accessible only to those directly involved in patient care. Data retention policies must respect both legal requirements and the intimate nature of the hospice environment.

Narratives from staff highlight the delicate balance between surveillance and respect. A hospice nurse recounted a patient who became agitated when a motion sensor inadvertently triggered a light while the family shared quiet reflection. The team immediately recalibrated the system, realizing that technological precision must never override emotional safety. These experiences underscore the need for staff to understand not only the technical functions of devices but also their human impact.

Technology must be unobtrusive. Devices should blend into the room's design rather than dominate it. Hidden sensors, recessed speakers, and integrated control panels maintain the room's aesthetic and emotional tone. When technology is visually prominent, it can remind patients of institutional oversight, undermining the sense of home and calm that hospice spaces strive to create.

Staff training is essential for ethical implementation. Caregivers must understand the ethical principles, technological functions, and potential emotional consequences. Competency includes knowledge of when to override automated systems, how to communicate device usage to families, and how to troubleshoot unexpected issues without disrupting care rituals.

The principle of proportionality guides ethical decisions. Only technologies that serve a clear, demonstrable purpose—safety, comfort, or ritual facilitation—should be introduced. Devices that offer marginal benefit but carry significant intrusion risk should be avoided. This principle helps maintain trust between staff, patients, and families.

Narratives further illuminate the emotional dimensions of technology. One hospice aide described a patient who rested more peacefully knowing that fall alerts were silently active, without the constant presence of staff. The patient reported feeling "protected but not watched," highlighting the potential for technology to enhance dignity when implemented thoughtfully.

Equity is an ethical concern. Technologies must be accessible to all patients, regardless of socioeconomic background, cultural identity, or spiritual preference. Systems that privilege certain families, languages, or cultural practices risk exacerbating inequities in emotional and ritual support. Inclusive design ensures that ethical standards extend beyond technical function to social fairness.

Integration with existing human-centered care is critical. Technology should act as a supporting actor, not as a replacement for human presence. Automated systems can handle mundane tasks, reminders, or monitoring, freeing staff to focus on bedside presence, relational care, and ritual facilitation. When technology substitutes for human interaction, ethical boundaries are compromised.

Staff reflections reveal that ethical dilemmas are often situational. The same monitoring system that provides comfort in one case may provoke anxiety in another. Teams must continually assess patient responses, family feedback, and situational appropriateness. Ethical practice is therefore dynamic, not static.

Confidentiality extends to family interactions as well. Audio and video systems should never inadvertently capture conversations outside the scope of care. Staff must ensure that personal discussions, spiritual counseling, or familial expressions of grief remain private, reinforcing trust in the hospice environment.

Temporal ethics are also relevant. Data should be used only for immediate care needs or ritual facilitation. Long-term storage of intimate information without explicit consent raises significant ethical questions. Clear policies on data life cycle, access, and deletion are necessary to uphold dignity.

In emergency situations, ethical principles remain guiding. Technology may be activated to prevent harm, but staff must continue to balance safety with emotional space. Rapid interventions should minimize intrusion and communicate care intentions clearly to families and patients whenever possible.

Cultural and spiritual sensitivity informs ethical use. Devices that support ritual must be customizable to accommodate diverse practices. A system designed to play prerecorded prayers, for example, must allow families to select content that aligns with their spiritual or cultural framework, avoiding assumptions or defaults that may unintentionally offend.

Technology can enhance shared decision-making. Families often find reassurance when they can visualize or understand how devices function. Transparent communication about purpose, limitations, and ethical safeguards builds trust and reinforces collaborative care.

Staff training should include debriefing protocols after sensitive incidents. When technology fails or triggers unexpected responses, ethical reflection and discussion support continuous improvement. Teams can refine system use while honoring patient dignity and emotional safety.

Case narratives highlight the psychological benefit of ethical technology. Families describe a sense of security when monitoring systems are clearly explained and discreetly implemented. Patients report comfort in knowing staff remain attentive without feeling constantly observed, demonstrating the synergy between ethics, technology, and human care.

Ultimately, ethical technology in hospice transforms the room into a supportive, respectful space. Devices act as silent allies—monitoring, signaling, and guiding ritual—without diminishing human presence. The ethical framework ensures that technology reinforces compassion rather than compromising it, maintaining the hospice mission of dignity, comfort, and relational care.

Ethics in technology reminds us that no system exists in isolation. Each sensor, speaker, or automated light must be evaluated in the broader context of emotional architecture, ritual practice, and family experience. When these factors are harmonized, technology becomes a seamless participant in a human-centered hospice ecosystem, enhancing care without intruding on intimacy.

10

Education, Staff Training, and Design Translation

Orientation in hospice begins long before patient care—it begins with the environment itself. For new staff members, understanding the intentional design of each room is foundational. Room layout, sightlines, and material choices are not merely aesthetic decisions; they are carefully calibrated tools that influence patient perception, family engagement, and the rhythm of rituals.[1] Teaching caregivers to recognize these subtleties ensures that their interactions complement the architecture rather than inadvertently disrupt the delicate emotional balance within the room.

Architectural literacy is the first essential skill for new staff. During orientation, they are introduced to the purpose behind every spatial element: why beds are not immediately visible from the door, how window placement invites reflection, and how circulation paths minimize emotional and physical disruption. Recognizing this choreography allows caregivers to perform essential clinical tasks while preserving the serenity of the space, demonstrating that movement within the room can itself be a form of caregiving.

Materials are taught not as decorative flourishes but as tactile and psychological instruments. Wood paneling, matte surfaces, and soft textiles convey warmth and invite touch, reinforcing the patient's sense of comfort and identity.[2] Staff learn how these choices facilitate connection: Patients may instinctively reach for a warm wooden table, a soft blanket, or a textured chair arm, reinforcing the room as a space of safety and intimacy.

Story-based training is central to spatial orientation. New nurses and aides hear narratives of prior patients and families that illustrate how room features facilitated or impeded ritual, vigil, or intimacy. A story may recount how a chair by the window became a locus of reflection during long vigil hours, teaching staff the invisible significance of furniture placement and its capacity to frame emotional experience. These stories bridge theoretical knowledge with practical understanding.

Orientation emphasizes sightlines and visual cues. Staff are instructed on which angles allow observation without intrusion, which perspectives preserve dignity, and how subtle repositioning can maintain calm during clinical interventions. Visual training includes learning how light interacts with textures, how furniture arrangement signals sacred zones, and how unbroken sightlines can enhance both family rituals and staff efficiency.

Lighting is introduced as both a practical and emotional tool. Staff learn how to manipulate dimmers, bedside lamps, and shading devices to complement ritual or emotional tone. They are taught to read the room's natural light cycles, understand the interplay of sunlight with materials, and employ artificial light strategically. Proper lighting enhances comfort, signals sacred time, and helps families intuitively understand transitions without verbal guidance.

Sound awareness is another pillar of orientation. Staff are trained to move quietly, minimize cart noise, and respect the acoustic properties of the room.[3] Voice modulation is emphasized, teaching staff how whispered conversations, gentle storytelling, or soft instructions can maintain a serene environment. Orientation also addresses sound sequencing, ensuring that patients and families experience a calm, predictable auditory environment.

Scent integration is introduced with subtlety. Staff learn how olfactory cues—diffusers, herbal infusions, or ritual incense—interact with memory and emotional presence. Training emphasizes moderation and cultural sensitivity, ensuring scents enhance ritual or care moments without overwhelming the senses. Awareness of smell becomes a complement to other sensory dimensions of the room, reinforcing the multisensory approach to hospice care.

Staff are trained to recognize "micro-zones" within each room: the bedside vigil zone, the reflection zone by the window, the staff zone near clinical tools, and the memory zone where personal objects are displayed.[4] Understanding these zones allows caregivers to navigate the room with purpose, preserving intimacy, supporting rituals, and maintaining emotional coherence. This zoning knowledge also reduces stress by giving staff a mental map of where interactions are most appropriate.

Orientation also includes emergency adaptability. Staff learn to rearrange furniture for family gatherings, spiritual ceremonies, or clinical interventions without compromising the room's intended emotional atmosphere. These exercises underscore that flexibility is not merely practical but deeply ritualistic, allowing for continuity of care in unpredictable circumstances while maintaining the sanctity of space.

Narratives about patient positioning highlight spatial significance. For example, a nurse recounts guiding a family to sit in particular areas during vigil hours, relying entirely on visual and spatial cues rather than verbal instruction. These narratives demonstrate how attentive observation and environmental understanding can facilitate profound nonverbal communication between staff, patients, and families.

Observation exercises allow new staff to experience the effects of room design firsthand. Trainees shadow experienced nurses, noting how furniture arrangement, lighting, and object placement influence family behavior and patient comfort. Reflection sessions afterward encourage staff to articulate insights and recognize the subtle choreography of space in action, integrating experiential learning with architectural theory.

Staff orientation emphasizes sensory sequencing. Caregivers learn to orchestrate light, sound, and scent to create a predictable emotional rhythm. For instance, dimming lights while introducing a gentle aroma signals vigil hours, enabling families to understand transitions intuitively. This training fosters the development of rhythm-conscious caregiving, in which environmental cues guide emotional experience.

Cultural competence is embedded in spatial training. Staff learn how architectural elements support diverse spiritual and cultural rituals, from directional bed placement to movable furniture and accessible surfaces for ritual objects. Orientation emphasizes respecting these accommodations while ensuring caregiving remains seamless and unobtrusive.

Documentation protocols are integrated into orientation. Staff are trained to record family preferences, environmental adjustments, and ritual practices. This ensures continuity across shifts and reinforces the room as a medium for memory and presence. Accurate documentation allows incoming staff to honor existing rituals and maintain emotional coherence within the room.

Ethical considerations are highlighted from the start. Staff are taught to balance technology with dignity, ensuring nonintrusive monitoring, privacy, and autonomy. Orientation emphasizes that technological tools—lighting automation, subtle sound systems, and discreet monitoring devices—should blend seamlessly into the environment, supporting care without overshadowing human interaction.

Hands-on practice is a cornerstone of orientation. Trainees manipulate lighting, sound, furniture, and other room elements to observe how small adjustments affect family behavior, patient comfort, and ritual flow. Experiential learning ensures that staff internalize principles that cannot be fully communicated through lectures or manuals alone.

Mentorship reinforces these lessons. Experienced staff model spatial sensitivity, demonstrating how subtle gestures, movement paths, and furniture adjustments preserve serenity and emotional continuity. Observing mentors in action allows trainees to internalize practices, creating a culture of attention and reverence for the environment.

Feedback is incorporated systematically. Trainees provide reflections on how room features influenced their ability to support rituals, maintain dignity, and manage emotional presence. This iterative approach reinforces staff awareness, encourages personal reflection, and aligns behavior with the architecture's intended emotional outcomes.

Finally, orientation instills respect for the room as a living archive. Staff are taught that each patient leaves an emotional imprint on the space, and their actions contribute to that legacy. Understanding that they are both caretakers and stewards of memory reinforces the hospice philosophy: Continuity, compassion, and human-centered design are inseparable from the built environment.

Embedding ritual knowledge begins with understanding that hospice care is not only clinical but also profoundly symbolic. Every act, from a warm washcloth to the subtle dimming of a lamp, conveys care, presence, and emotional continuity. Staff must internalize these micro-rituals to support families and patients in ways that are both tangible and spiritually resonant.

Training starts with the warm washcloth ritual, a practice that goes beyond hygiene. Staff learn to fold, heat, and present the cloth in a manner that communicates respect and comfort. The tactile warmth conveys a sense of safety and personal attention, creating a nonverbal message of dignity.[5] Trainees practice slow, deliberate motions that allow the patient to feel attended to without anxiety.

The handholding ritual is emphasized next. Staff are taught to offer handholding at critical moments: during vigil hours, transitional care, or final breaths. Orientation focuses on positioning, grip, and duration, acknowledging that physical touch communicates reassurance more powerfully than words alone.[6] Families often learn this behavior intuitively by observing staff, reinforcing the social transmission of care.

Lamp dimming serves as both practical lighting control and emotional cue. Staff are trained to adjust light levels gradually, signaling transitions such as vigil commencement or quiet reflection. This ritualized use of lighting provides temporal structure, giving both patients and families a nonverbal understanding of sacred time within the room. Staff practice these adjustments alongside stories that illustrate the emotional significance of light modulation.

Memory surface arrangement is another critical element. Trainees learn to curate bedside tables, shelves, and small altars without cluttering the space. Placing photos, trinkets, or symbolic objects requires attention to aesthetics, cultural significance, and family preference. Staff are taught that these surfaces serve as both memory anchors and emotional guides for grieving families. Families, in turn, often mirror these arrangements, intuitively learning to participate in the ritual of presence.

Staff practice integrated ritual choreography, combining these elements into fluid sequences. For example, while dimming the lamp, they might offer a warm cloth, hold a patient's hand, and adjust a memory surface. This simultaneous attention to multiple ritual layers teaches caregivers to move seamlessly through the room, preserving serenity and reinforcing continuity for both patient and family.

Case studies are a key component of ritual training. One narrative describes staff creating a personalized family ritual for a patient whose children wanted to participate in the vigil. Staff guided them in arranging objects, timing handholding, and selecting soft background music. The family learned by observing and imitating, while the patient experienced a tailored, emotionally resonant environment.

Staff are trained to observe family cues for participation. Orientation emphasizes that rituals are co-created; families often intuitively adopt gestures and timing from staff behavior. Caregivers are taught to step back, allowing the family to take the lead while providing gentle guidance, ensuring rituals are meaningful and culturally aligned.

The sequence of care is central to embedding ritual knowledge. Staff practice routines that integrate hygiene, touch, memory, and environmental cues into a cohesive flow. This teaches them that each ritual act has temporal significance, supporting the patient's emotional and physiological comfort while reinforcing the sacred character of the space.

Verbal framing complements physical ritual. Staff learn soft phrasing, tone modulation, and timing of words to accompany gestures. A simple "I'm here with you" during handholding, or a whispered story while adjusting the memory surface, enhances the emotional impact and models ritual behavior for families.

Orientation emphasizes sensory layering. Staff are trained to integrate touch, light, sound, and scent in ways that communicate continuity. For example, dimming a lamp while releasing a gentle lavender aroma reinforces the start of vigil hours. This multisensory orchestration creates a cohesive, emotionally supportive environment that guides families intuitively.

Cultural competence is central to embedding ritual knowledge. Staff are taught to recognize and honor diverse traditions, from prayer rituals and song to object placement and hand gestures. They learn to adapt micro-rituals without diminishing their symbolic value, ensuring all families feel included and respected.

Staff practice mindful observation, learning to recognize subtle signs of comfort or distress. This allows real-time adjustment of ritual gestures—handholding duration, memory surface arrangement, or lighting changes—to respond to patient and family needs. Such responsiveness reinforces the perception of ritual as living, adaptive, and personal.

Reflection sessions follow practical training. Staff discuss observed outcomes, sharing stories of moments in which ritual had profound impact. For example, one family observed a nurse adjusting a chair by the window while dimming lights and offering a memory object; they later mirrored this behavior themselves, learning the ritual nonverbally.

Ritual reinforcement extends across shifts. Staff are trained to document family preferences, successful sequences, and environmental adjustments. This ensures continuity and prevents the erosion of carefully established emotional routines, allowing rituals to persist even when staff change.

Staff are taught the symbolic layering of space, understanding that each object, gesture, and environmental cue contributes to an overarching narrative. Even seemingly minor acts—smoothing a blanket or repositioning a chair—carry ritual weight and communicate presence, dignity, and continuity.

Orientation includes scenario-based training, in which staff practice responding to unexpected situations while preserving ritual integrity. For instance, a sudden medical intervention requires temporary modification of light, touch, or object placement while maintaining emotional continuity for families.

Observation of experienced mentors is emphasized. New staff shadow seasoned caregivers, witnessing the seamless integration of ritual into care. Mentors verbalize reasoning behind gestures, environmental adjustments, and family guidance, providing a bridge between theory and embodied practice.

Staff are encouraged to develop ritual intuition, internalizing sequences so that actions are performed fluidly and empathetically. This ensures that gestures become second nature, allowing focus on the patient and family rather than on mechanical procedure.

Feedback loops reinforce learning. Staff reflect on how rituals impacted family engagement, patient comfort, and room atmosphere. This iterative process encourages refinement of technique, attentiveness, and sensitivity to cultural and emotional nuances.

Finally, embedding ritual knowledge emphasizes that staff are co-creators of the emotional architecture. Each gesture, touch, and environmental adjustment contributes to a continuum of care, memory, and presence. Staff learn that mastery of micro-rituals transforms the hospice room from a clinical space into a living, sacred environment in which families can grieve, connect, and honor the life that has passed.

Architect–staff collaboration is the essential bridge between theoretical design and lived experience, ensuring that hospice spaces are not only functional but also emotionally attuned. This collaboration transforms static blueprints into responsive environments in which care, ritual, and memory coalesce seamlessly. Without this partnership, spaces risk prioritizing aesthetics or efficiency over the nuanced needs of patients, families, and staff.

The collaboration typically begins with orientation tours in which architects walk through hospice units alongside nurses, aides, and other frontline staff. These guided tours reveal subtle patterns of movement, furniture usage, and object placement that might never be captured in architectural plans. Staff provide real-time commentary, noting how bed placement, window views, or doorway alignments influence both patient dignity and family engagement during vigil hours.

Feedback loops form the backbone of ongoing collaboration. Staff routinely report their observations regarding lighting, sound, and spatial arrangements. Architects interpret these insights and propose design adjustments. This iterative process transforms the environment into a living laboratory, in which small modifications—such as moving a chair or adjusting a lamp—can have profound effects on ritual continuity and emotional comfort.

Lighting adaptation is a frequent area of focus. Staff may observe that a bedside lamp casts shadows across a patient's face during evening vigil hours, inadvertently reducing the intimacy of family interactions. Architects respond by repositioning fixtures or providing tunable lighting controls, allowing staff to modulate illumination in ways that preserve both dignity and emotional resonance.[7]

Furniture ergonomics also benefits from collaborative observation. A chair that appears aesthetically pleasing may, in practice, be uncomfortable for prolonged family use. Architects adjust armrest height, seat depth, and cushioning to accommodate long vigil hours, ensuring both family comfort and staff functionality, while maintaining the room's aesthetic harmony.

Soundscapes are continually refined through collaboration. Staff report that distant hallway noise, beeping monitors, or rolling carts disrupt the sanctuary of a hospice room. Architects work with acoustic consultants to integrate sound-absorbing panels, carpeting, and subtle masking technologies, ensuring that the room's auditory environment aligns with emotional needs.

Case studies illustrate the value of iterative adjustments. In one hospice, staff noted that a bedside table's location interfered with ritual arrangements. Architects reconfigured the table and added modular storage, allowing families to place memory objects, photos, or symbolic items without obstruction. The result was a tangible improvement in ritual fluidity and family engagement.

Observation of human behavior informs every design decision. Architects watch how staff move through spaces, carry equipment, and interact with families. These observations guide the placement of essential items such as call buttons, linen carts, and hand hygiene stations, minimizing intrusive movement while preserving serenity.

Narratives from staff provide qualitative data that cannot be captured through metrics alone. A nurse might describe repositioning a chair to allow better visibility of a patient's hand during a final farewell. Architects translate these stories into practical design guidelines, demonstrating how intimate observations influence architectural choices.

Iterative prototyping ensures that designs meet both functional and emotional requirements. Mock-ups of furniture, lighting, or memory surfaces are tested in situ. Staff provide feedback on usability, comfort, and emotional impact, and designers refine prototypes until the environment supports both care and ritual seamlessly.

Technology integration is another area enriched by collaboration. Sensors, dimmable lights, and sound systems are evaluated in real-life scenarios. Staff indicate which features are intuitive, unobtrusive, and emotionally supportive, guiding architects in selecting technology that enhances care without overshadowing the human experience.

Emergency protocol observations guide design adjustments to accommodate rapid changes. Architects witness staff responding to sudden patient distress and adjust layouts or access points to enable quick intervention without disturbing family presence or ritual continuity.

Cultural and spiritual considerations are essential. Staff report how various religious or cultural practices—directional bed placement, object arrangement, or ritual sounds—interact with spatial design. Architects embed flexibility into layouts, ensuring that rooms can accommodate diverse spiritual and familial practices without privileging one tradition.

Training in spatial literacy is integrated into collaboration. Staff learn to recognize design cues—light gradation, sightline clarity, and furniture placement—as part of their daily caregiving routines. Architects, in turn, gain insight into unspoken behavioral patterns that influence how space is experienced.

Narrative reflections document successes and challenges over time. Stories of families interacting with memory surfaces or light rituals inform both design refinements and training materials. These qualitative accounts serve as living evidence of the environment's impact on emotional and ritual outcomes.

Cross-disciplinary workshops create shared understanding. Architects, nurses, and aides participate in scenario-based exercises, exploring how interventions such as light adjustment, object placement, or sound modulation affect care dynamics. These exercises strengthen the collaborative relationship and improve practical outcomes.

Material selection is informed by staff feedback on tactile and emotional responses. Caregivers report which surfaces feel warm, inviting, or calming. Architects integrate these insights while balancing durability, maintenance, and aesthetic integrity, ensuring materials support ritual, care, and patient comfort simultaneously.

Temporal design adjustments are guided by staff observation. Families and patients respond differently to changes in light and sound throughout the day. Architects adjust lighting schedules, window treatments, or sound cues to align perceived temporal rhythms with emotional needs, subtly structuring care and reflection.

Continuous observation is institutionalized through digital logs or journals. Staff record successes and challenges, providing architects with ongoing feedback. This approach ensures that design remains a living, adaptive system responsive to the evolving needs of patients, families, and staff.

Integration of sensory pathways—including light, sound, scent, and touch—is constantly refined. Staff indicate how combined stimuli influence comfort, alertness, or ritual engagement. Architects fine-tune placements and intensities to create holistic, emotionally coherent environments.

Ethical collaboration considers both autonomy and dignity. Staff input helps architects ensure that monitoring technologies, lighting automation, or sound systems enhance care without imposing on patients' or families' privacy. The environment becomes a silent facilitator of respect and presence.

Ultimately, architect–staff collaboration transforms hospice spaces into living, responsive sanctuaries. By blending empirical observation, narrative reflection, and iterative design, the team ensures that architecture itself participates in caregiving. Spaces evolve continuously, honoring both the practical and emotional dimensions of end-of-life care, supporting families and staff while preserving the sanctity of the patient's experience.

Hospice care is inherently dynamic, and the environments that support it must evolve in tandem with both patient needs and staff practices. Continuous learning and adaptation create a living, iterative cycle of observation, feedback, and refinement, allowing physical spaces to remain sensitive to emotional, ritualistic, and practical demands over time. Spaces are not static; rather, they are responsive entities that absorb human activity and shift subtly to accommodate rituals, comfort, and dignity.

The process often begins with story collection. Staff routinely record observations, noting how families respond to furniture arrangements, lighting, soundscapes, or memory surfaces. These qualitative narratives capture emotional and behavioral cues that standard clinical documentation may overlook, offering invaluable insight into how the physical environment interacts with human presence and ritual.

Observation-based learning is a cornerstone of adaptation. Multidisciplinary teams, including architects, nurses, and social workers, conduct structured walkthroughs of patient rooms. They examine how families engage with the space at different times of day, noting, for instance, that morning sunlight enhances a memory surface but may cast harsh shadows across a seating area. These insights inform minor adjustments in furniture placement, blind control, or lamp orientation, with profound effects on emotional tone and practical usability.

Staff reflections further enrich the learning process. Caregivers note patterns of comfort or distress and link these to environmental triggers. A nurse might observe that a humming heating unit disturbs patients during vigil hours, prompting a mechanical adjustment or the introduction of soft masking sound to restore tranquility. Such small interventions can dramatically improve patient and family experiences.

Multidisciplinary meetings institutionalize these observations into actionable change. Nurses, social workers, chaplains, facility managers, and architects gather regularly to review environmental feedback. These sessions encourage cross-disciplinary problem-solving and ensure that decisions honor both functional requirements and emotional needs. For example, a minor repositioning of chairs might alleviate congestion for families while preserving sightlines to ritual spaces.

Case Example

In one hospice unit, staff reported that memory surfaces by windows often became cluttered, interfering with rituals and sightlines. Architects responded by introducing modular shelving units and defined display areas, allowing families to personalize spaces without creating visual chaos. This adjustment enhanced both practical use and emotional resonance.

Iterative modification is central to continuous learning. Changes are intentionally small, reversible, and carefully documented. Adjusting a lamp angle, repositioning a chair, or relocating a memory object may seem minor but can significantly influence how families engage with the space. Over time, these cumulative adjustments create a refined, emotionally attuned environment.

Staff training evolves alongside architectural changes. Caregivers are oriented to new layouts, lighting schemes, or soundscapes, with instruction emphasizing the emotional rationale behind each change. This ensures that staff behavior remains aligned with design intentions, reinforcing the integration of architecture and caregiving.

Observation of family behavior provides further data. Staff note movement patterns, preferred seating, and object interaction. These observations influence future room arrangements, ensuring that spaces support both intuitive and structured use.[8] A chair that initially obstructed a window might be repositioned to offer a better view, fostering contemplation and vigil practice.

Environmental audits complement anecdotal observations. Architects and staff assess light levels, sound intensity, and air quality to ensure technical standards support emotional and ritual needs. These audits may reveal subtle stressors, such as background noise or glare, that interfere with comfort and care.

Feedback integration combines formal surveys, anecdotal reports, and direct observation into a central system that architects and staff reference when proposing adjustments. This ensures that environmental interventions reflect lived experiences rather than theoretical design principles.

Narrative insight drives empathetic design. Stories of families connecting with a memory surface, or patients soothed by diffused light, inform decisions that purely technical assessments cannot justify. Architecture thus becomes responsive to human emotion as much as to physical function.

Continuous learning extends beyond individual rooms. Hallways, common areas, and transition spaces are observed to maintain emotional continuity. Staff identify areas where incidental noise, poor acoustics, or visual clutter might disrupt the calm atmosphere, prompting design or behavioral adjustments.

Trial and observation cycles allow modifications to be tested incrementally. For example, a new dimming schedule for vigil hours may be implemented in one room and monitored for several weeks before wider adoption. This careful, evidence-informed approach reduces unintended consequences while enhancing comfort.

Ritual observation is crucial. Micro-rituals—blanket repositioning, lamp dimming, or object placement—are monitored to assess how environmental changes enhance or impede these practices. Adjustments are made to support a range of cultural and personal rituals without enforcing a rigid template.

Design responsiveness balances competing priorities. Enhancing sightlines for family observation may compromise privacy if not carefully considered. Continuous learning emphasizes negotiation and compromise, informed by repeated observation and staff insight.

Documentation is meticulous. Every adjustment, rationale, and observed outcome is recorded, forming a living record of the environment's evolution. These records are essential for staff orientation, longitudinal study, and knowledge transfer to new hospice teams.

Technology integration is evaluated within this adaptive framework. Automated lighting, climate control, or sound systems are continually refined based on staff and family feedback. Adjustments, such as slower dimming sequences or scent diffusion schedules, are calibrated to support rituals without intrusion.

Cultural sensitivity is woven into adaptation. Changes are evaluated for alignment with spiritual practices, family traditions, and individual preferences. Flexible design ensures that spaces remain inclusive, accommodating diverse customs without imposing uniformity.

Professional development is reinforced through feedback loops. Staff become skilled observers of environmental cues, learning to identify subtle stressors and comfort indicators. This observational skill enhances caregiving quality and fosters a culture of reflective practice, linking professional identity with spatial awareness.

Ethical reflection is embedded in adaptation. Staff and designers consider the emotional, cultural, and spiritual consequences of each environmental change. Adjustments are made with mindfulness toward patient autonomy, family needs, and ritual integrity, ensuring ethical consistency in a highly intimate context.

Narrative reflection closes the loop. Stories of comfort, emotional release, or ritual success provide qualitative validation of changes, guiding subsequent refinements. Each positive response reinforces design principles and informs staff practices.

Ultimately, continuous learning and adaptation transform hospice spaces into living, responsive environments. Through iterative feedback, multidisciplinary collaboration, and attentive observation, architecture becomes an active participant in care, supporting emotional continuity, ritual integrity, and a sanctuary of presence for patients and families alike.

Hospice environments exist at the intersection of deeply human care and strict regulatory oversight. Policies and accreditation standards provide necessary frameworks to ensure patient safety, infection control, accessibility, and staff accountability. However, these frameworks can sometimes appear at odds with the subtle, emotionally attuned architectural and ritual practices that define high-quality end-of-life care. Navigating this intersection requires thoughtful integration, ensuring that regulatory compliance complements rather than undermines the emotional environment.

The first principle in aligning design with policy is understanding how regulatory codes translate into spatial requirements. Fire safety, exit accessibility, ventilation, and infection control standards dictate certain minimum parameters, such as aisle width, window height, and materials used. Architects and staff must collaborate to interpret these codes in ways that preserve dignity and flexibility within the room.

Case Example

A hospice team faced strict infection control rules that mandated impermeable surfaces near patient beds. Rather than relying on cold, glossy finishes that reminded patients of hospital wards, designers opted for matte, antimicrobial-treated wood and textile blends that satisfied safety regulations while preserving sensory warmth. This creative approach ensured compliance without sacrificing comfort or ritual usability.

Staff training in policy awareness is critical. Nurses, aides, and volunteers are educated on how accreditation standards influence the environment, from electrical safety to hazardous material storage. This knowledge helps caregivers understand why certain materials or arrangements exist, allowing them to work within the rules while still prioritizing emotional and ritual needs.

Administrative observation reveals the benefit of embedding design awareness into policy adherence. Leaders note that staff who understand both the safety rationale and emotional intention behind design principles are more confident and less likely to create improvisations that could undermine either safety or ritual integrity.

Narrative Insight

In one unit, a family expressed concern about the placement of a memory shelf near the window. Staff explained the infection control and fire code considerations behind the fixed installation, and then demonstrated how the shelf could still serve as a personal shrine. The family was reassured, and the room maintained both compliance and emotional resonance.

Accreditation standards—such as those from the Joint Commission or state-specific hospice regulations—often emphasize documentation, traceable procedures, and environmental risk mitigation. Designers and administrators translate these standards into practical elements without disrupting the quiet, reflective atmosphere. For instance, emergency pull cords are integrated discreetly into furniture design, ensuring accessibility without visual intrusion.

Balancing privacy and policy is a recurring theme. Health Insurance Portability and Accountability Act (HIPAA) and confidentiality standards require visual and auditory barriers, but these must be implemented in ways that do not make families feel segregated or the space clinical. Strategically placed curtains, sound-absorbing partitions, and sightline-conscious furniture provide this balance.

Case Example

A new unit required reinforced exits for safety compliance. The design team preserved sightlines from family chairs to the patient bed while incorporating the required doors and alarms. The result was a secure space that remained emotionally legible and comfortable.

Documentation protocols intersect with design-informed practice. Staff record environmental checks—such as light levels, sound levels, and memory surface arrangements—as part of routine safety audits. These records simultaneously satisfy regulatory requirements and reinforce the principles of emotional architecture.

Infection control integration often challenges textural and material choices. Soft textiles, memory objects, and rugs carry emotional and ritual significance but must be cleanable or removable for hygiene purposes. Teams develop cleaning schedules and modular object placement to maintain both emotional warmth and compliance.

Policy-driven flexibility is also important. Accreditation often requires certain fixed measurements and spatial configurations, but careful design allows modularity elsewhere in the room. Folding chairs, mobile sound diffusers, and adjustable lighting enable the room to adapt to family size, rituals, and patient needs while still meeting mandated standards.

Staff reflections frequently emphasize that compliance and compassion are mutually reinforcing rather than mutually exclusive. A nurse may note that following hand hygiene or ventilation standards gives families confidence in the care environment, which in turn enhances trust and emotional openness.

Technology compliance must also integrate into the emotional environment. Automated monitoring, call systems, and smart environmental controls are designed not just for efficiency but also for alignment with privacy, data security, and safety codes. The technology remains invisible, supporting care without violating regulatory norms.

Narrative Insight

An administrator recounted that the adoption of accreditation-aligned lamp dimming protocols allowed both compliance with electrical standards and preservation of ritual lighting for evening vigil hours. Families appreciated the subtle consistency, reinforcing a sense of reliability and calm.

Environmental hazard mitigation often intersects with ritual behavior. Candles and incense are prohibited in many facilities; flame-free LED alternatives and scent-safe diffusers ensure that ritual practices can continue safely. Staff are trained to supervise these rituals in accordance with fire and safety codes.

Training reinforcement occurs through routine simulations and audits. Staff practice responding to emergencies, maintaining hygiene, and adhering to infection control procedures while preserving the emotional integrity of the space. These exercises embed compliance behavior into habitual care practices.

Policy evolution can benefit from staff and architectural feedback. Accreditation bodies may allow for design exceptions if compelling evidence demonstrates that emotional or ritual considerations improve care outcomes. Administrators document these cases, creating a precedent for future facility designs.

Continuous observation loops ensure that regulatory compliance evolves alongside practice. Teams regularly review room layouts, object placement, and material durability to confirm that safety and emotional design goals remain aligned as rituals, technology, and family expectations shift over time.

Ethical alignment is central to policy integration. Caregivers consider the balance between rule-following and compassionate practice, ensuring that adherence to regulations enhances—not detracts from—the dignity, privacy, and emotional well-being of patients and families.

Case Example

In one hospice, alarm systems were adjusted to comply with emergency code without startling families during vigils. Staff documented the adjustment and noted improvements in patient restfulness and family perception of care quality.

Ultimately, embedding policy and accreditation knowledge into hospice practice ensures that emotional architecture, ritual fidelity, and operational safety coexist harmoniously. By framing regulations as a scaffolding rather than a limitation, teams create spaces in which families feel secure, patients experience dignity, and staff are empowered to act confidently within a compliant yet human-centered environment.

Epilogue

In the quiet of a hospice room, silence is not empty; it is an active participant in the choreography of care. Every surface, every fold of linen, every flicker of light contributes to a delicate ecosystem in which human presence, ritual, and architecture converge. The walls are not inert barriers—they absorb the weight of whispered conversations, the cadence of labored breaths, and the soft footsteps of those who come to witness, to grieve, or simply to be. In this space, time itself seems malleable, stretching and contracting according to the rhythm of life's final hours.

The bed, positioned with care away from the doorway, functions as both a literal and symbolic center. It holds the patient's body while simultaneously serving as a stage for presence, ritual, and reflection. Families naturally orient themselves around it, forming concentric circles of support, each movement and gesture imbued with meaning. Caregivers move with intention, their steps choreographed to honor both physical and emotional comfort, allowing the bed to become a locus of dignity and devotion.

Light is not merely functional; it carries emotional resonance. Tuned to the needs of patients and families, it signals transitions, marks the beginning of vigil hours, and frames moments of intimacy and reflection. The gentle dimming of a bedside lamp becomes a ritual itself, a visual cue that invites pause, reverence, and awareness. In this orchestration, light dances alongside human presence, guiding attention and lending depth to otherwise ordinary spaces.

Objects within the room acquire significance far beyond their practical purpose. A favorite mug, a well-worn blanket, or a photograph of a life lived become anchors of presence, grounding both the patient and the family in memories and continuity. Each object is intentionally curated, a tangible manifestation of love, identity, and ritual. These items carry stories forward, providing tactile and visual reminders of a life intertwined with the space.

The vigil chair by the window serves as more than a piece of furniture; it is a throne of devotion. Families spend long hours seated here, observing breath, listening to whispered memories, and silently bearing witness. The window frames the external world, allowing the patient and family to perceive the passage of time, weather, and light, connecting the intimate interior to the vastness of nature beyond. From this vantage, the chair becomes a metaphor for both watching and letting go, a bridge between life and memory.

Textiles and material choices communicate care without words. Linen sheets, weighted blankets, and woven throws encourage touch and closeness, inviting hands to hold, arms to embrace, and hearts to remain open. The textures of wood, ceramic, and matte surfaces create an environment that is tactile, grounding, and emotionally supportive, offering reassurance through material presence as much as human interaction.

Sound is orchestrated with the same intentionality as light and material. Silence is protected, yet layers of gentle sound—nature's rustle, the timbre of human voice, and the subtle chime of ritual—offer a framework for emotional orientation. Noise control is not purely practical; it is ethical, acknowledging the fragility of life and the necessity of providing a sanctuary for those in transition.

Scent threads through the room as an invisible narrative. Lavender, cedar, or familiar home aromas trigger memory, reduce anxiety, and anchor the spirit. Ritualized scent, whether through essential oils, flame-free incense, or herbal infusions, marks temporal transitions, signaling moments of reflection, prayer, or closure. These olfactory cues harmonize with light, sound, and object arrangement to create a fully immersive and comforting environment.

Technology, when present, is subtle, supportive, and invisible. Automated lighting, climate control, discreet sensors, and virtual presence tools do not intrude; they enhance the orchestration of care, allowing families to focus on presence and connection while maintaining patient safety. Technology becomes an unobtrusive partner in the architecture of compassion, ensuring that human interaction remains central.

Staff rituals—pausing after a patient passes, resetting the room, smoothing blankets, or placing a symbolic token—intertwine with architectural intention. These repeated actions build continuity and emotional resonance, transforming the room into a living archive of care. Through ritual, the staff honors both the patient and their own emotional experience, sustaining resilience and professional identity.

Family rituals emerge organically, guided by the room's design. Folding a blanket, arranging photographs, or whispering a story becomes a meaningful act within the spatial and temporal framework of the room. These gestures are not random; they are embedded within the architecture itself, creating a choreography of love and presence that honors the patient's life.

Memory lingers in the room, both visible and invisible. Walls, furniture, and surfaces retain traces of past care—gestures, touch, and stories left behind. Spatial memory informs future interactions, offering comfort to those who enter, even if the history is not consciously known. This invisible community binds families and staff across time, a living repository of human experience.

Time behaves differently within these spaces. The usual cadence of life slows, allowing moments to stretch, breaths to deepen, and attention to settle.

Architecture, light, and ritual shape the perception of time, creating a rhythm that honors both patient and family, allowing presence to flourish without the constraints of the outside world.

Flexibility and adaptability are essential. Rooms expand and contract to accommodate varying numbers of visitors, cultural rituals, or spiritual practices. Movable furniture, modular surfaces, and adaptable lighting respond to the unpredictable, ensuring that the space serves the needs of every patient and family, facilitating rituals without disruption.

Natural elements provide grounding and continuity. Views of gardens, plants, water features, and seasonal light cycles link the interior to the rhythms of the world outside. Nature softens the perception of pain, reduces stress, and mirrors the emotional arc of care, creating a holistic experience that aligns the internal and external environments.

The hospice room is more than a container; it is an active partner in the process of caregiving. Every architectural choice—from proportion to material selection, from lighting to sound control—reflects intentionality. Each decision communicates respect, reverence, and dignity, reinforcing the human-centered purpose of the space.

Education ensures that staff understand the significance of space and ritual. Through orientation, narrative-based learning, and continuous reflection, caregivers learn to inhabit the room with sensitivity, awareness, and confidence. This integration of knowledge and practice preserves the integrity of both care and design, ensuring consistent, compassionate interaction.

Policy, compliance, and accreditation are seamlessly integrated into design. Safety, hygiene, and ethical standards are embedded within the room's architecture, supporting both functional and emotional needs without compromising the sanctuary's sanctity. Care and regulation exist in harmony, enabling both dignity and safety.

The room is a vessel for stories, for grief, and for gratitude. Each life leaves an imprint, shaping the experience of subsequent occupants. Chairs creak differently, light falls at familiar angles, and surfaces bear the memory of gentle hands. These echoes are not haunting but sacred, creating an environment that nurtures reflection, care, and emotional resilience.

Every death transforms the room. Objects remain temporarily, scents linger, and lights dim in deliberate ritual. The space mediates transition, preserving the continuum between life and memory. It honors the patient, supports the family, and sustains staff through practices that carry meaning and reverence.

Presence, ritual, and design converge to teach a profound lesson: that even at the end of life, creativity, attentiveness, and compassion endure. The room becomes a teacher, illustrating how space, material, light, sound, scent, and technology can harmonize to foster dignity and connection.

Families leave the room carrying not only memories of their loved one but also an imprint of the space itself: the textures, smells, sounds, and light that shaped their experience. These sensory residues become part of the grief process, offering comfort, guiding reflection, and providing continuity for memory and mourning.

The quiet room demonstrates that architecture is never neutral. Every choice—whether spatial, material, or technological—affects human experience profoundly. In hospice, where attention to presence and ritual is paramount, design becomes a moral as well as aesthetic imperative.

As the door closes softly behind the departing family and the bedside lamp is dimmed for the last time, the room exhales. Its silence is rich, layered with traces of love, care, ritual, and human presence. It is both archive and witness, repository and sanctuary, holding within it the essence of human transition.

Ultimately, the hospice room is a blueprint for compassionate design. It teaches that architecture can serve as a partner in care, preserving dignity, honoring ritual, and sustaining both families and caregivers through life's final chapter. In this room, care is composed, presence is preserved, and quiet is a living, breathing testament to humanity.

References

Chapter 1

1. Ulrich, R. S., et al. (2008). Evidence-based healthcare design. *HERD: Health Environments Research & Design Journal, 1*(3), 61–125.
2. Ulrich, R. S. (1984). View through a window may influence recovery from surgery. *Science, 224*(4647), 420–421.
3. Waller, S., & Finn, H. (2017). Healing spaces: The science of place and well-being. *Journal of Dementia Care Design, 5*(2), 12–18.
4. Vartanian, O., et al. (2016). Impact of ceiling height on the experience of interior space. *Journal of Environmental Psychology, 46*, 103–115.
5. Chalmers, A., & Gallichio, K. (2020). Entrances, thresholds, and transition spaces in palliative care. *Palliative Architecture Review, 2*(1), 44–59.
6. Lawson, B. (2010). *Healing architecture.* Architectural Press.

Chapter 2

1. Cajochen, C. (2016). Effects of light on human circadian rhythms, sleep and mood. *Somnologie, 20*, 193–201.
2. Porter, G., Leonards, U., Troscianko, T., Haworth, J., Bayer, A., & Tales, A. (2012). Dealing with illumination in visual scenes: Effects of ageing and Alzheimer's disease. *PLoS ONE, 7*(9), e45104. https://doi.org/10.1371/journal.pone.0045104
3. Veitch, J. A., & Newsham, G. R. (2018). *Lighting quality and energy-efficiency effects on task performance, mood, and health in offices.* National Research Council of Canada.

Chapter 3

1. Byock, I. (2014). *The four things that matter most.* Atria Books.
2. Rosenblatt, P. C. (2000). *Parent grief: Narratives of loss and relationship.* Routledge.
3. Pallasmaa, J. (2012). *The eyes of the skin: Architecture and the senses.* Wiley.
4. McNamara, B. (2001). *Fragile lives: Death, dying and care.* Open University Press.
5. Turner, V. (1969). *The ritual process: Structure and anti-structure.* Aldine.

Chapter 4

1. Waldrop, D. P., & Meeker, M. A. (2012). Communication and the care of people with dementia and terminal illness: Foundations of ritual, touch, and sensory comfort. *Journal of Palliative Care, 28*(3), 160–168.
2. Back, A. L., et al. (2009). *Mastering communication with seriously ill patients: Balancing honesty with empathy and hope.* Cambridge University Press.
3. Kagawa-Singer, M., Blackhall, L. J., & O'Neill, S. (2015). Cultural approaches to end-of-life care: Ritual, meaning, and the built environment. In: A. Alpers, B. Lo, & C. Sandborg (Eds.), *Cross-Cultural Medicine* (pp. 189–216). Philadelphia, PA: American College of Physicians.

Chapter 5

1. Ulrich, R. S. (1999). Effects of healthcare environmental design on medical outcomes. *Journal of Healthcare Design, 11*, 97–109.
2. Pallasmaa, J. (2012). *The eyes of the skin: Architecture and the senses.* Wiley.

3. Caspari, S., Eriksson, K., & Naden, D. (2015). The meaning of space for family members in hospice care. *Journal of Clinical Nursing, 24*(3–4), 579–588.
4. Boyce, P. R. (2014). *Human factors in lighting*. CRC Press.
5. Blauert, J. (1997). *Spatial hearing: The psychophysics of human sound localization*. MIT Press.
6. Kellehear, A. (2014). *The inner life of the dying person*. Columbia University Press.
7. Bachelard, G. (1964). *The poetics of space*. Beacon.

Chapter 6

1. Ulrich, R. S., et al. (2008). A review of the research literature on evidence-based healthcare design. *HERD: Health Environments Research & Design Journal, 1*(3), 61–125.
2. Graham, J., & Barter, J. (2021). Cultural and spiritual considerations in end-of-life architecture: Designing for diversity. *Journal of Palliative Care Design, 5*(2), 14–29.
3. Joseph, A. (2006). *The impact of the environment on infections in healthcare facilities* (Issue Paper No. 1). Center for Health Design.

Chapter 7

1. Ulrich, R. S., et al. (2008). A review of the research literature on evidence-based healthcare design." *HERD: Health Environments Research & Design Journal, 1*(3), 61–125.
2. Livingston, G., et al. (2020). Dementia: The Lancet Commission Report. *Lancet, 396*(10248), 413–446.
3. van den Bosch, K. A., et al. (2020). The effects of environmental sound on patients' health outcomes: A systematic review. *Applied Acoustics, 164*, Article 107259.
4. Evans, G. W., & McCoy, J. M. (1998). When buildings don't work: The role of architecture in human health. *Journal of Environmental Psychology, 18*(1), 85–94.
5. Annerstedt, M., et al. (2013). Inducing physiological stress recovery with sounds of nature in a virtual environment. *Physiology & Behavior, 118*, 240–250.
6. Ratcliffe, E., et al. (2013). Bird sounds and their contributions to perceived attention restoration and stress recovery. *Journal of Environmental Psychology, 36*, 221–228.

Chapter 8

1. Herz, R. S. (2016). The role of odor-evoked memory in psychological and physiological health. *Brain Sciences, 6*(3), Article 22.
2. Lillehei, A. S., & Halcon, L. L. (2014). A systematic review of the effect of inhaled lavender on sleep quality. *Holistic Nursing Practice, 28*(1), 64–74.
3. Howard, S., et al. (2020). Aromatherapy and perceived relaxation: A mixed-methods study using lavender essential oil. *Complementary Therapies in Medicine, 53*, Article 102534.
4. Buckle, J. (2015). *Clinical aromatherapy: Essential oils in healthcare* (3rd ed.). Elsevier.
5. Kim, J. T., et al. (2011). The effect of lavender aromatherapy on preoperative anxiety in ambulatory surgery patients. *Journal of Alternative and Complementary Medicine, 17*(8), 823–826.
6. Harvey, G. (2011). *Indigenous religions: A companion*. Bloomsbury.
7. Ballard, C. G., et al. (2002). Aromatic essential oils and enhanced cognitive function in dementia. *International Journal of Geriatric Psychiatry, 17*(12), 1123–1127.

Chapter 9

1. Bakker, R., & Ijzerman, H. (2019). Circadian lighting in healthcare environments: Effects on patient well-being and caregiver stress. *Journal of Environmental Psychology, 66*, Article 101338.
2. Chan, A. H. S., et al. (2020). Automation and cognitive load in healthcare environments. *Ergonomics in Design*, 28(3), 10–18.
3. Zhang, H., & Arens, E. (2021). Thermal comfort among vulnerable populations: Implications for end-of-life care. *Building and Environment, 200*, Article 107973.

4. Ulrich, R. S. (2019). Environmental stress reduction through multisensory cues in health facilities. *Health Environments Research & Design Journal, 12*(4), 42–56.
5. Ferris, F. D., & Bruera, E. (2018). Environmental and psychosocial contributors to terminal agitation. *Palliative Medicine, 32*(6), 1045–1051.
6. Wang, C., et al. (2020). Non-contact vital sign monitoring in palliative and acute care. *IEEE Reviews in Biomedical Engineering, 13*, 79–98.
7. Stevenson, D. G., & Russell, D. (2019). Acoustic considerations in hospice and palliative care design. *HERD: Health Environments Research & Design Journal, 12*(3), 122–137.
8. Gipson, K., et al. (2021). Predictive monitoring for comfort optimization in end-of-life care. *Palliative Care Research, 34*(2), 145–157.
9. Moore, J., & Caudill, P. (2022). Digital presence and family connectedness in hospice care. *Journal of Palliative & Supportive Care, 20*(1), 65–72.
10. World Health Organization. (2021). *Telehealth in palliative care: Ethical and design guidelines.*
11. Krebs, L. (2018). Multisensory design strategies in palliative rituals. *Journal of Hospice & Palliative Nursing, 20*(6), 514–520.
12. Thompson, G., & Chochinov, H. M. (2020). Ritual and environmental modulation in end-of-life settings. *Palliative & Supportive Care, 18*(4), 451–459.

Chapter 10

1. Ulrich, R. S. (2001). Effects of healthcare environmental design on medical outcomes. In: A. Dilani (Ed.), *Design & Health: The Therapeutic Benefits of Design* (pp. 49–59). Stockholm: Svensk Byggtjänst.
2. Daykin, N., Byrne, E., Soteriou, T., & O'Connor, S. (2008). The impact of art, design and environment in mental healthcare: A systematic review of the literature. *Journal of the Royal Society for the Promotion of Health, 128*(2), 85–94.
3. National Consensus Project for Quality Palliative Care. (2018). *Clinical practice guidelines for quality palliative care* (4th ed.).
4. Verderber, S. (2003). *Innovations in hospice architecture.* Routledge.
5. Field, T. (2010). Touch for socioemotional and physical well-being: A review. *Developmental Review, 30*(4), 367–383.
6. Goldstein, P., et al. (2018). Brain-to-brain coupling during handholding. *Proceedings of the National Academy of Sciences, 115*(11), E2528–E2537.
7. Figueiro, M. G., & Rea, M. S. (2010). The effects of light on human health and behavior: Implications for lighting design in healthcare settings. *Journal of Healthcare Engineering, 1*(1), 1–22.
8. Hamilton, D. K., & Watkins, D. H. (2009). *Evidence-based design for multiple building types.* Wiley.

Index

For the benefit of digital users, indexed terms that span two pages (e.g., 52–53) may, on occasion, appear on only one of those pages.

A

accent lighting, 22, 23, 26, 29, 31, 32, 81, 83, 85, 92

acoustics, 1, 4, 5, 10, 16, 66, 68, 69, 74, 77, 80, 82, 83, 86, 91

adaptability, 81, 83, 84–87, 91

agency, patient, 8, 17, 35, 37

air quality, 81, 84, 87, 89

alarms, 101, 103, 126, 127, 128, 135

alcoves
- clinical, 6
- conversation, 15
- memory, 6, 17
- reflection, 6

ambient lighting, 21, 26, 30, 32

architecture
- active role of, 4, 17
- behavioral ecology and, 14–17
- as caregiver, 90–91, 92
- dignity and, 4, 5, 8, 9, 17, 79, 81, 82, 84, 92
- emotional architecture of light, 18, 21, 24, 33
- as ethical act, vii
- hospice care and, 1, 5
- memory-supportive architecture, 70–73
- as participant in care, 4, 17
- ritual-centered architecture, 90
- stillness and, 1
- thresholds and, 8–11
- as witness, 5, 76, 78, 84, 92

archives
- hospice room as, 65, 67–68, 70, 76, 78

B

bed placement
- dignity and, 5, 7
- emotional orientation and, 2
- threshold visibility and, 5, 8–9

behavioral ecology, 15–16, 17

biophilic design, 87–90, 92

blankets
- emotional resonance of, 34, 37, 44–45, 46, 47
- weighted blankets, 45, 46

boundaries
- emotional containment and, 15
- personalization boundaries, 71, 73

brightness
- emotional modulation through, 18, 19, 27

C

candles
- cultural ritual use of, 28, 33
- ritual candles, 36, 38, 40

caregiving
- architecture supporting, 79, 82, 84, 90–91
- caregiving rituals, 51–53
- environmental support for, 3, 15–16
- light as caregiving instrument, 21, 30, 33

chairs
- bedside placement of, 5–6
- reflection chairs, 66, 72, 74, 75, 77
- vigil chairs, 41–44
- window chairs, 41–44

circadian rhythms, 2, 7, 18, 20–21, 24, 25, 26, 27, 67, 73–74, 75, 88, 90

clinical cues
- concealment of, 3, 10

clocks
- battery removal rituals, 48, 49, 50
- emotional symbolism of, 47–50
- ticking clocks, 47–48

clutter
- emotional overload and, 70, 71, 72
- memory without clutter, 70–73

color palettes
- earth tones, 4
- muted palettes, 4

comfort
- environmental comfort and, 1, 4–5
- tactile comfort and, 12, 13

compassion
architecture as, 5, 11
material compassion, 4
continuity
environmental continuity, 3, 10
narrative continuity, 35, 36–37, 39–40
relational continuity and ritual, 51, 52, 53, 56, 58, 64
temporal continuity and clocks, 48–50
visual continuity, 13
cultural rituals, 53, 54, 59–62, 66–67, 69, 79, 81, 83, 86, 90, 92

D
daylight
circadian orientation and, 19, 24–27
emotional grounding and, 25, 26
death rituals
final breath ritual, 62
transition rituals, 62–64
dignity
architecture and, 4, 5, 8, 9, 17, 79, 81, 82, 84, 92
body care and, 62–63
illumination and, 18, 20, 21, 28, 30–31, 33
object placement and, 34, 35, 37, 40
dimming rituals, 27–30

E
emotional architecture, 4, 21–24, 67–68, 70, 73, 76, 79, 81, 84, 90
emotional regulation
lighting and, 18–19, 20–21, 31–32, 33
rituals as regulators and, 52, 56, 58
environmental psychology, 2, 18, 21, 53, 56, 57, 65, 69, 70

F
families
emotional regulation and, 4–5
illumination and, 19, 20, 22, 27, 28–29
movement through zones, 8
spatial orientation and, 7
family rituals
hand-holding circles, 54
journaling rituals, 54, 56
night-watch rituals, 54
permission rituals, 54
storytelling rituals, 54, 55, 56
farewell rituals, 22, 27, 28, 32
flexibility
adaptable hospice rooms and, 81, 83, 84–87, 91, 92
flooring
acoustic flooring, 4, 13, 14
quiet flooring and, 80, 82, 83, 87

G
geometry
calming geometry, 1–2
soft geometry and, 79, 81–82
glow pockets, 22, 23, 29, 31, 32
grief
containment of, 4, 15
grief processing and spatial memory, 70, 76, 77
object-mediated grief support, 34–35, 37, 39, 40, 47

H
hallways
hospice contrast with, 3, 8, 10
healing environments
biophilic healing and, 87–90
hospice rooms
emotional atmosphere of, 1, 18–21
future hospice room design, 90–92
sanctuary quality of, 4–5, 11

I
identity
personal identity through objects, 35, 36–37, 39–40, 46
ritual preservation of identity, 51, 54, 55
illumination
emotional function of, 18, 21, 30–33
layered illumination and, 21–24
indirect lighting, 2, 9, 11, 19, 21, 22, 23, 25, 27, 79–80, 83, 85, 88, 91
intimacy
lighting and relational closeness, 19, 22, 27, 31–32
object-supported intimacy, 35–36, 37, 45
spatial permission for, 15

L
layered illumination
ambient-task-accent model, 21–24, 26, 32
light
as emotional instrument, 18, 21, 30, 33
as physiological regulator, 18, 20–21, 24, 25, 26, 27
lighting
accent lighting and ritual, 61, 63
adaptive lighting systems and, 21, 24, 29–30, 33

programmable lighting systems and, 21, 23, 24, 29–30, 81, 85, 90
ritual lighting and, 53, 55, 60, 62
listening
architecture as, vii
design as, viii

M
materials
emotional resonance of, 11–14
interaction with light and, 20, 25
natural materials and, 79, 80, 82, 83, 85, 87, 89, 91, 92
tactile qualities of, 11–14
memory
illuminated memory objects and, 23, 29, 31, 33
memory anchors, 70, 71, 75, 76, 77
memory surfaces, 38–40, 71, 72, 73, 77, 80, 83–84, 86, 90, 91, 92
narrative memory and objects, 36, 39–40, 46, 50
spatial memory, 65–68
temporal memory and, 73–76
micro-rituals
caregiving micro-rituals, 51–53
silent micro-rituals, 53
movement
caregiver movement, 3, 7–8
intuitive movement pathways and, 79, 80, 82, 87
unobstructed movement, 6, 11
multisensory design
sensory integration and, 81, 82, 86, 87–90

N
nature
emotional grounding through, 3–4, 8–9, 10
nature as co-designer, 87–90
views to nature and, 81, 87, 88–90
night lighting
low-level illumination and, 20, 22, 26

O
objects
emotional anthropology of, 36
objects as anchors of presence, 34–38
objects as ritual instruments, 35
ritual objects and, 55, 57–58, 60, 61, 63, 64, 66–67, 75, 77, 79, 80, 83–84, 86, 89, 90, 91, 92
symbolic objects, 34, 36–37, 38, 48
orientation
emotional orientation, 7, 8, 11
temporal orientation, 18, 19, 20, 23, 24, 26, 27

P
patina, 12–13, 44, 65, 67, 74
presence
anchored through objects, 34, 35, 36, 37–38, 40
environmental support of, 4, 14, 17
ritualized presence and, 51, 52, 53, 56, 64
vigil presence and, 41–44
privacy
threshold privacy and, 1, 5
privacy through sightline management, 84, 86, 90

Q
quiet
architectural quiet, 1, 4–5
sound reduction and, 1, 4
quiet rooms
definitions of, vii
future-oriented quiet room design, 90–92
purpose of, vii
sanctuary function of, 4–5, 11

R
reflection
lighting and contemplative space, 22, 26
reflective ritual practices and, 52, 53, 54, 55
vigil reflection and, 41–44
reflection zones, 6, 7, 17, 80–81, 82, 88, 89, 92
rituals
body-care rituals, 62–63
caregiving rituals, 51–53
clock rituals, 48, 49
cultural and spiritual rituals, 59–62
family rituals, 53–56
object-as-ritual, 35
transition rituals, 62–64

S
sacred space
rituals creating sacred space, 57, 60, 62
vigil chairs and, 41
sacred time
dimming light and, 27, 30
transition rituals and, 59, 61, 62
sanctuary
hospice room as, 65, 73, 76, 78, 81, 84, 88, 92
illumination and sanctuary atmosphere, 22, 27

sensory grounding
  tactile grounding through objects, 36, 45
  warm washcloths and touch rituals, 51, 52
  weighted blankets and, 45
sensory regulation, 2–3, 17
sightlines
  clutter-free sightlines, 1–2, 79, 80, 81–82, 84, 86, 91
  layered sightlines, 9–10
  threshold sightlines, 8, 11
silence
  architecture of silence, 1
  as care, vii
  engineered silence and, 80
  ritual silence and, 55, 56–57, 62, 63, 64
  as spatial condition, vii
sound
  acoustic buffering, 1, 10
  sound absorption, 1, 13, 16
soundscapes
  biophilic soundscapes and, 85, 86, 88, 90, 91
  hospice soundscapes and, 68, 69, 74, 77
  ritual soundscapes and, 55, 60–61, 63
spatial coherence, 7, 8, 15, 67, 71, 73
storytelling
  memory objects and, 36, 39–40, 49, 50
  ritual storytelling and, 54, 55, 56, 58
stress reduction
  environmental stress reduction, 2, 4–5, 17
  warm lighting and, 18, 20–21, 23–24, 30

T
tactile comfort, 12, 13
temporal architecture
  hospice temporal design and, 73–76
textiles
  comfort textiles, 44–47
  weighted textiles, 45, 46
thresholds
  cultural meaning of, 9, 10
  emotional transition and, 8–11
  first impressions and, 8–9, 11
  lighting at, 9, 11
  sound buffering at, 10
transition rituals
  post-death transition rituals, 62–64

V
ventilation
  natural ventilation, 87, 89
  quiet ventilation systems and, 81, 84, 87, 89
vigils
  family vigils and, 53, 54–55, 58
  lighting and, 19, 21, 25, 27
vigil zones, 5–6, 7, 17, 80–81, 82, 85, 86, 89, 91
vulnerability
  architecture and, 2, 5
  illumination and emotional vulnerability, 18, 21

W
warm lighting
  emotional safety and, 18, 19, 20, 22, 27, 31–32
warm washcloth ritual, 51, 52
water features
  fountains and auditory calm, 88, 89, 90, 91, 92
weighted blankets, 45, 46
windows
  biophilic window placement and, 79, 80, 81–82, 84, 87, 88–89, 91
  daylight orientation and, 19, 24–25, 26
  emotional grounding and, 3–4, 5, 6–7, 13
  opening windows after death, 62
  vigil chair placement and, 41, 42, 43
witness
  architecture as witness, 5, 76, 78, 84, 92
  clocks as witnesses, 48, 50
  collective witness and, 53, 54, 56, 57–58, 64
  light as witness to ritual and grief, 21, 30
  room as witness, 76, 77, 78
  vigil chairs as witness spaces, 41, 42, 44